Psychology for Nursing & Healthcare Professionals

Developing Compassionate Care

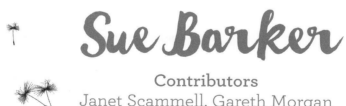

Sue Barker

Contributors
Janet Scammell, Gareth Morgan
Andrew Santos, Beverley Johnson
Gemma Stacey-Emile & Hamed Al Battashi

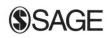
SAGE

Los Angeles I London I New Delhi
Singapore I Washington DC I Melbourne

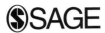

Los Angeles | London | New Delhi
Singapore | Washington DC | Melbourne

SAGE Publications Ltd
1 Oliver's Yard
55 City Road
London EC1Y 1SP

SAGE Publications Inc.
2455 Teller Road
Thousand Oaks, California 91320

SAGE Publications India Pvt Ltd
B 1/I 1 Mohan Cooperative Industrial Area
Mathura Road
New Delhi 110 044

SAGE Publications Asia-Pacific Pte Ltd
3 Church Street
#10-04 Samsung Hub
Singapore 049483

Editor: Becky Taylor
Editorial assistant: Charlène Burin
Production editor: Katie Forsythe
Marketing manager: Camille Richmond
Cover design: Wendy Scott
Typeset by: C&M Digitals (P) Ltd, Chennai, India
Printed and bound by CPI Group (UK) Ltd,
Croydon, CR0 4YY

Library of Congress Control Number: 2015959799

British Library Cataloguing in Publication data

A catalogue record for this book is available from
the British Library

ISBN 978-1-4739-2505-2
ISBN 978-1-4739-2506-9 (pbk)

At SAGE we take sustainability seriously. Most of our products are printed in the UK using FSC papers and boards.
When we print overseas we ensure sustainable papers are used as measured by the PREPS grading system.
We undertake an annual audit to monitor our sustainability.

Contents

About the Authors

Sue Barker is a lecturer in Mental Health at Cardiff University; she has been a mental health nurse for over 30 years and is a chartered psychologist and Associate Fellow of the British Psychological Society. She has always been concerned with emotional well-being and her PhD focused on emotional care. Her phenomenological approach to understanding people's emotional experiences has supported her teaching and writing related to person-centred, humanised and compassionate care.

Gemma Stacey-Emile qualified as a mental health nurse just over 20 years ago; she has spent most of her time working in the field of substance misuse and more recently joined Cardiff University as a lecturer at the School of Healthcare Sciences. As well as her interest in substance misuse, Gemma has a keen interest in leadership and management and enjoys teaching these subjects at the School. She is also interested in helping others utilise their own personal skills to help motivate others to provide high standards of care.

Gareth Morgan is a lecturer in Research Methods, Ethics and Policy at Cardiff University; he has been a lecturer for over 25 years and is a qualified social worker. As such, he has always been interested in the human condition and the influence of wider structures on people's lives. He currently lectures primarily in Allied Health and, in particular, has contributed to the development and ongoing evolution of the Occupational Therapy programme. He also manages the associate lecturer scheme at the School of Healthcare Science, which supports the secondment of health professionals to the School for a prescribed period.

Hamed Al Battashi is a lecturer in Mental Health at Oman Specialized Nursing Institute, based in Muscat, Sultanate of Oman. He is a certified counsellor and a member of the Honor Society of Phi Kappa Phi at the Villanova University Chapter, USA. He is also a certified trainer in thinking skills and developing creativity. He has always been interested in exploring human relationships and the impact of cultures in influencing people's perceptions and interactions with the world around them. His background as an educator has always motivated him to explore the role of the humanities in improving teaching experiences and enhancing students' learning. These interests have positively shaped his working attitude and his dealings with the people around him.

Janet Scammell is Associate Professor in Nursing at Bournemouth University. After a career in various roles in adult clinical nursing practice, Janet moved to higher education where she has specialised in nurse education for 25 years. She is a Principal Fellow of the Higher Education Academy. Her doctoral studies concerned internationally recruited nurses and their role as mentors to nurse students. Janet is a mentor for Mary

Seacole Award Scholars who focus on improving health outcomes for minority ethnic communities. Janet's areas of interest include practice-based learning, equality and diversity issues, humanising care for all but in particular for older people, and humanising healthcare professional education.

Beverley Johnson graduated from Oxford Brookes in 1994 as an adult nurse. She has worked in healthcare in Oxford, London, Australia and Cardiff. Beverley became a lecturer at Cardiff University in 2004 and has primarily taught Sociology and the Social Policy of Health. She is a lead for adult field nursing and is involved in the development and support of staff and students. She is interested in emotional well-being and emotional intelligence and is keen to develop knowledge and understanding of how they can enhance care provision and patient experience.

Andrew Santos is a lecturer at Cardiff University and a lead for adult nursing. As part of this role, he has responsibility for supporting both staff and undergraduate nurses. Alongside his academic role, he continues to work on a one-to-one basis with people who have complex health needs. He is committed to compassionate person-centred care.

Publisher's Acknowledgements

The publishers would like to thank the following lecturers for their invaluable feedback on the proposal and chapters:

Mark Arnold, London South Bank University, UK

Aimee Aubeeluck, University of Nottingham, UK

Thomas Beary, University of Hertfordshire, UK

Dr Kim Goode, University of Hertfordshire, UK

Lena Wiklund Gustin, Mälardalen University, Sweden

Dr. Julie MacInnes, Principal Lecturer, Canterbury Christ Church University, UK

Siobhan McCullough, Queen's University Belfast, UK

Linda Robson, Edge Hill University, UK

The publishers would also like to thank Jennie Barker for her fantastic illustrations, as well as Alex Oldham, Amy Scott and Imogen Fox for providing case studies. The book is much richer for your contribution.

The author and publishers are grateful to the following for their kind permission to reproduce material:

Table 4:1 is adapted from Department of Health (2012) *Compassion in Practice*, © Crown copyright 2012, Available at www.england.nhs.uk/wp-content/uploads/2012/12/compassion-in-practice.pdf

Table 4.4 is adapted from Gilbert, P. (2009) 'Introducing compassion-focused therapy', *Advances in Psychiatric Treatment*, 15:199–208. Reproduced with permission of The Royal College of Psychiatrists.

Table 10:2 Two sets of managerial styles is adapted from Bass, B.M. (1985) *Leadership and Performance beyond Expectations*. New York: Free Press, with permission of John Wiley and Sons.

Foreword

It is a privilege for me to write a foreword to this book because the concept of compassion is central to nursing practice and very close to my heart. I have been a nurse for 20 years and if you were to ask me what nursing is, I would firstly describe what nurses need to be like. Put simply, nursing is an evidence-based health practice of human kindness within a professional context. It is impossible to separate the practice of nursing from the qualities of the people who deliver the practice. I am going to start with a bold statement: Nursing is the second most important job in the world (I shall reveal the first, most important, at the end of my foreword!).

Over the years, nursing has become increasingly technical. As the profession has developed, it has rightly become closely allied to medical and health sciences. Nursing uses science, but it is primarily an art. I would argue that the art of nursing is often overshadowed by the dominance of science. In any discipline it is hard to reconcile arts and science and it is understandable that students may pay greater attention to science in their studies because science is often considered to be easier to learn than art. However, with every patient interaction, the nurse is practising his or her own art. Knowledge of all the nursing science in the world will not make a person a good nurse. Conversely, being a kind person is not enough to successfully deliver good nursing practice. However, unless the nurse understands the nature of the art of nursing, scientific knowledge alone is useless. So what is this art? It is certainly not a-theoretical. On the contrary, there are many theories and approaches that may help and instruct nursing practice and this is what this book delivers. The art of nursing is similar to the art of any human endeavour: it comes with theoretical knowledge and it comes with practice. This is recognised by regulatory bodies; usually, half of all nurse education is based in university classrooms and the other half is based in clinical areas. Together, a syllabus seeks to help the person develop from a lay-person to a professional under expert instruction.

This book draws a great deal from the discipline of psychology. This is a good (scientific) starting point for the art of nursing, because the 'good' nurse is primarily aware of psychological processes. Firstly, self-awareness is required – the study of one's own psychology. Next, the 'good' nurse needs understanding of other people, and finally what is needed is understanding of the complexities of human relationships. All of this then underpins what nurses do. As such, the nurse needs emotional intelligence as well as any other form of intelligence. If you would like to study this concept further, I would encourage you to read an article called 'The heart of the art: Emotional intelligence in nurse education' (Freshwater and Stickley, 2004). The idea for the need for compassion in nursing is essentially the need for emotional intelligence. The reason nurses need compassion is because human beings are not machines. Nurses are constantly working with people, often in pain or in emotional distress, and many we work with are coming towards the end of their lives. In nursing we often refer to person-centred care; this is essentially compassion in practice.

However, nurses are not angels! Being compassionate in a busy and demanding job is hard, especially when resources to do the work are often depleted. Compassionate nursing takes its toll and it is hard to maintain that emotional integrity when we are feeling exhausted, exploited and surrounded by pain and suffering. This book acknowledges what it is like to be a nurse in the real world and the toll it takes, and offers ways of managing, coping and hopefully thriving in the future.

This is a vital book for nurses today and I especially recommend it to all nursing students, who will learn a great deal by studying its pages. This only leaves me to identify the most important job in the world, which is of course being a parent.

Theo Stickley
University of Nottingham

Reference

Freshwater, D. and Stickley, T. (2004) 'The heart of the art: Emotional intelligence in nurse education', *Nursing Inquiry*, 11 (2): 91–98.

Introduction

About this book

Each chapter in this book presents a topic area to support compassionate care. We believe that in order to undertake compassionate care, there is a need for a psychological understanding of the person and their social as well as structural world. Throughout the book, there is recognition that compassionate care and those providing it are immersed in the prevailing culture – the cultural hegemony. Whilst the contemporary hegemony demands the provision of compassionate care, it does not always provide the necessary resources. The book therefore concludes by exploring how both well-being and compassionate care can be maintained.

Book structure

The book starts with an introduction to the major psychological approaches to understanding people. Chapter 1 offers a basic exploration of what psychology is and the main theoretical categories within it, and also provides a basic understanding of how psychologists develop their knowledge and research techniques. Chapter 2 uses the psychological theoretical categories along with the philosophical underpinnings to examine human development through the lifespan. Chapter 3 considers the nature of suffering because suffering can be seen to underlie the need for compassionate care. Chapter 4 discusses compassionate care in detail: what it is and why it is necessary.

Chapter 5 enables a deeper understanding of the phenomenon of compassionate care through an exploration of person-centred approaches, with their philosophical origins and contemporary issues being scrutinised in this area. Chapter 6 looks at the individual giving compassionate care and how psychological theory can help us understand ourselves and others. Chapter 7 unpacks the therapeutic tools available to us to provide care. Chapter 8 provides an explanation of the psychological theories supporting the skills that caregivers need. Chapter 9 identifies the impact that providing compassionate care may have on the individual and how they can maintain well-being.

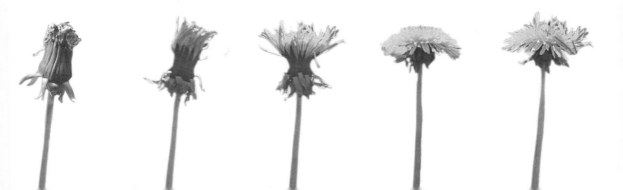

In Chapter 10, there is an implicit acceptance of the philosophies, psychological theories and research – already highlighted in the book – which are important in understanding and providing compassionate care. This last chapter considers how this can be sustained.

Learning features

There are a number of features to support your learning in this book. The text leads you through the main psychological theories in a particular topic, which are further explored and elaborated on through case studies so that you can see how these relate to care. These case studies are from care students, informal caregivers and health and social care academics. Some chapters have boxes where the theory is explained in more detail to facilitate greater understanding without disturbing the narrative of the relationship between care and theory.

Throughout the book, you will find activities aimed at helping you make sense of the theories. Some activities ask you to reflect on your own experiences, particularly those of caregiving and receiving. As these reflections are personal, no suggested answer is provided. Other questions ask you to think critically about a concept, theory or the application of a theory. These questions have outline answers provided at the end of the relevant chapter.

All the activities require you to take a break from reading, and think about the text and how it might support your care practice. At the end of each chapter, there are some suggested websites that you could access to further explore the given topic. Some of the websites are based on psychology but others focus more on the application of understanding, giving examples and providing video links.

1 Introduction to Psychological Theory

Sue Barker

I experience, I feel; I am human

I notice your suffering, I feel your suffering; I am sympathy

I sense your suffering, we share your suffering; I am empathy

Your pain is my pain, your comfort is my comfort; we share kindness

Together we are compassion!

Learning objectives

This chapter will introduce five perspectives of psychology and will explore how these perspectives offer differing understandings of the way people think, feel, behave and interact with others and their environment. These perspectives provide a basis for the subsequent chapters in order to develop a psychological understanding of compassionate care as experienced by care practitioners so as to enhance their performance of compassionate care. This chapter's learning objectives are to:

- Describe the five perspectives in psychology
- Identify a variety of research methods used in psychology
- Recognise the role of psychology in order to understand and explore care

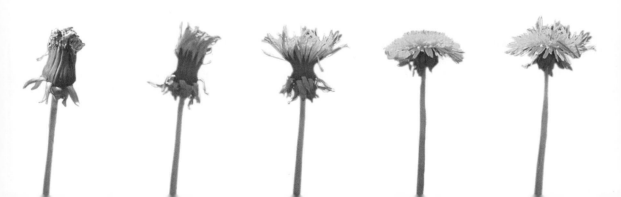

Activity 1.1   Critical thinking

Take a few minutes to consider why an understanding of psychology might be useful in your development of your caring skills.

Some suggestions are made at the end of the chapter.

Introduction

This chapter initially explores the five dominant psychological perspectives and considers how each of them may offer an explanation of caring practices. These will be referred to throughout the book. It will establish definitions of psychology and the research methods used to develop an understanding of people, particularly how and why they think, feel, behave and interact with others and how this differs between individuals. Research methods will be concisely described, identifying the major research approaches in psychology.

In order to explore any concept, a definition is required. So, despite psychology being explored throughout this book, an initial definition needs to be identified. I previously defined psychology in the following way:

> Psychology is a seeking to understand why people behave, think and feel the way they do, individually and in groups, in all areas of life including health. Psychologists seek not only to predict behaviour but also to change behaviours to enhance wellbeing and quality of life. (Barker, 2007: 2)

This is a simplistic definition but it can be used as a working definition. Many other authors have developed their own definitions but all have until recently been very similar, for example:

> Psychology is the study of behaviour and mental processes. Behaviour includes all of our outward or overt actions and reaction, such as talking, facial expressions and movements. Mental processes refer to all the internal, covert activity of our minds, such as thinking, feeling and remembering. (Ciccarelli and Myer, 2006: 4)

The most recent definition I could find, whilst identifying a focus on behaviour, extends my initial definition to include wider phenomenological experiences:

> The study of the nature, functions, and phenomena of behaviour and mental experience. The etymology of the word implies that it is simply the study of the mind, but much of modern psychology focuses on behaviour rather than the mind, and some aspects of psychology have little to do with the mind. (Colman, 2015: 724)

In the past, we have seen a move from philosophy exploring the nature of people through the Enlightenment and the development of scientific psychology to psychology stretching to include elements of philosophy. I believe that psychology (understanding people) and philosophy (the love of wisdom) have always been intimately related – and we are moving towards a greater acceptance of this.

Psychology has a number of different ways of trying to understand the person, which can support practitioners in their compassionate care practice. One of the methods used is termed **perspectives**. These perspectives have changed over the years but the most commonly used now are:

- Biological
- Psychodynamic
- Behavioural
- Cognitive
- Humanistic

Each of these perspectives has a different explanation or theory related to a person and their behaviour. These influence not only psychological understanding but also how this understanding can be developed (research) and applied to acts of care.

Biological psychology

Biopsychologists are often accused of **reductionism**, which means that they reduce the person by examining their individual biological components in order to understand them and their behaviour, instead of attempting to understand them as an **embodied** whole.

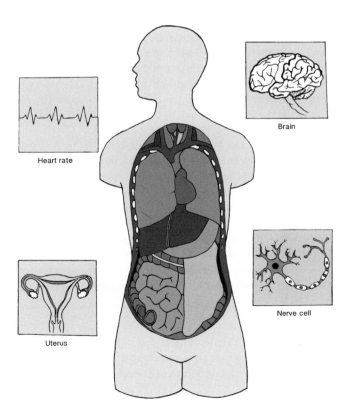

Figure 1.1   Sense of reduced body

Their explanations of human behaviours are through anatomical or physiological changes such as chemical reactions in the nervous and endocrine systems.

An understanding of biological functioning or the physiological influence on behaviour is important for most caring practitioners. Not responding to a physiologically produced behaviour could lead to death: for example, a person clutching their chest struggling to stand up, walk or talk may be having a 'heart attack' (myocardial infarction) which requires urgent attention.

Case study

 ## Miriam Walker – student nurse

I was asked to monitor the well-being of an elderly lady, Mrs Beverley Crosland, who had just been admitted to an assessment ward. Her husband was with her. Mrs Crosland appeared confused and agitated and she was saying she wanted to go home. Her husband was very worried. He said Beverley's concentration, attention and memory had deteriorated dramatically over the past week. Mrs Crosland was also groaning at times as if she was in pain. Whilst monitoring Mrs Crosland, her pulse rate appeared a little raised, along with her temperature, breathing and blood pressure. Mrs Crosland and her husband were unable to explain what they thought was wrong, although Mr Crosland implied he was concerned that his wife was developing dementia as he had heard about it on the television.

Despite my concerns, as the signs may have been indicative of dementia, I explained to both of them that I needed to ask a few more questions and she may need to have some tests before a decision could be made. Mr Crosland remained anxious and Mrs Crosland was becoming more confused with each question I asked.

At this point, I stopped following the assessment questions in the order they were set out and sat down next to Mrs Crosland rather than the other side of the table where I had been sitting to write down their answers. I passed the assessment questions to Mr Crosland and asked him to complete them as best he could. He appeared pleased to have a role to undertake and conscientiously started filling in the forms.

I then asked Mrs Crosland to tell me what she would like to be doing at the moment whilst holding her hand. She tried to think and then started to clutch her abdomen. I said 'Does your tummy hurt?' and I reached to touch her abdomen. I asked 'Do you need to go to the toilet?' She then said she could not go. I asked if Mr and Mrs Crosland thought she could be constipated and they both agreed she could be. They both were happy with a doctor conducting an examination to check.

After a physical examination, it was found that Mrs Crosland was constipated and she was offered an enema to allow some rapid relief. Mrs Crosland's agitation reduced and her mental functioning slowly returned to what was normal for her. She was also prescribed a laxative for a couple of weeks and given information on diet, exercise and her other medications.

In the case study of Miriam Walker, in which she believed she offered compassionate care, it can clearly be seen that what are understood to be psychologically important mental processes, such as attention, concentration and memory, are strongly influenced by biological functioning.

Biopsychologists, like human biologists, identify biological functions that produce certain behaviours but their focus is different to biologists. Biopsychologists seek to understand psychological issues: issues related to the mind or spirit. It could be said that the biopsychologists are interested in how biology supports and influences a person's thoughts, feelings and behaviour to produce individual differences whereas a biologist's focus is on describing or understanding the structure and function of the biological apparatus of the individual. Both can use an empirical, positivist, scientific approach to gaining knowledge (research).

Therefore biopsychologists and biologists explore the following but examine them through different 'lenses' – to use an optical analogy:

- Genes
- Anatomical differences
- Development through the lifespan
- Biological systems such as
    o The Nervous System
    o The Endocrine System

Biopsychologists explain behavioural change and individual differences through changes in the nervous system, endocrine system, or anatomical or genetic structure. There are numerous factors that could influence this functioning, such as:

- Development and maturation
- Infection
- Mutation
- Nutrition
- Disease
- Trauma
- Environmental factors

They suggest that people develop through a sequence of bodily maturation and growth determined by the endocrine and nervous systems. Therefore behaviour could be explained, in the absence of disorder or disease, by the maturational stage of development, genetic makeup, hormonal state and neural readiness (Barker, 2007). All of these will be influenced by environmental factors such as nutrition, stimulation, protection from disease, etc.

Genes

Each cell of the human body contains a nucleus. This nucleus usually has 23 pairs of chromosomes. These chromosomes contain the genetic code for the person and are composed of deoxyribonucleic acid (DNA). This genetic code provides the **genotype** for the person: the colour of their hair, their potential height, etc. What is seen of the person is said to be their **phenotype**, that is, the genotype that has been influenced by the environment.

Nervous system

There are two major parts in a human nervous system: the central nervous system (CNS) and the peripheral nervous system. The central nervous system is the brain and spinal cord; these are 'central', in the centre of the body. The peripheral nervous system is the large number of nerves surrounding the central system or at the outer limits of the body.

The peripheral nervous system has three parts:

- Cranial nerves (CN)
- Spinal nerves (SN)
- Autonomic nervous system (ANS)

All three (CN, SN, ANS) transmit information from the senses to the central nervous system and take commands from the central nervous system to various parts of the body. The cranial nerves link with the brain, the spinal nerves to the spinal cord, and the autonomic nervous system primarily controls the internal organs.

The autonomic nervous system can be further divided into three components:

- Sympathetic nervous system
- Parasympathetic nervous system
- Enteric nervous system

The sympathetic system prepares the body for action whereas the parasympathetic system prepares the body for rest. The enteric system regulates the digestive system and is influenced by both the parasympathetic and sympathetic nervous systems.

Endocrine system

The endocrine system is a collection of glands that secrete hormones into the body. The major endocrine glands are described in Table 1.1.

Biopsychologists study how each of these areas influence the behaviour of the person in their search to understand that behaviour. There is clear scientific evidence to support the theory that the nervous system and endocrine system communicate with each other. This is achieved through chemicals produced from these systems. Neurotransmitters (in the nervous system) influence the production of hormones (endocrine system) as nerves infiltrate the glands and hormones circulate in the body, thereby changing the chemical environment of the nerves.

Table 1.1 Endocrine glands and their principal effects

Gland	Principal effect
Pineal gland	Regulates seasonal changes and puberty
Hypothalamus	Regulates hormones released from the pituitary gland
Pituitary gland	Produces a number of hormones which stimulate growth and development
Thyroid	Involved in metabolism and blood homeostasis
Adrenal glands	Regulate metabolism and body hair. Help maintain blood sugar levels
Pancreas	Involved in the metabolism of sugars
Gonads	Stimulate the development and maintenance of sexual characteristics and behaviour

Source: Barker (2007: 6)

Summary of biopsychologists

Biopsychologists seek to understand individual behaviour using an **empirical, positivist,** scientific approach. They explain how people develop and how their behaviour changes through a maturational sequence as the nervous and endocrine systems develop to fulfil genetic encoding (genotype) or not (phenotype). The case study of Miriam Walker offers an understanding of the importance of care practitioners having a biological understanding of behaviour and behaviour change in order to allow them to offer appropriate care. We will find that other perspectives offer us an understanding of the importance of how we provide that care.

Activity 1.2   Reflection

Think of a time when you cared for someone and they appeared sad, unable to concentrate, found it difficult to organise themselves or were anxious. These are psychological 'symptoms'. Thinking back, did they have a physical health problem that might have caused these symptoms?

As this is a reflection, there is no outline answer at the end of the chapter.

Psychodynamic psychology

Introduction

This perspective in psychology relates to the theory developed by Sigmund Freud, but his dynamic theory of the mind has been adapted and developed by others since its inception. Theorists in this field include Alfred Adler, Erik Erikson and Carl Gustav Jung (students of Freud but by some considered neo-Freudians), along with Melanie Klein and Anna Freud.

Freud lived from 1856 to 1939 and his work has become a significant part of both psychological and Western societal thinking. Freud had a classical education that included philosophy. He studied at the Brentano School at the same time as Edmund Husserl (see Chapter 5) and both view the mind as having psychic energy. Freud went on to study medical science and was particularly interested in neurology but later trained in clinical medicine, became a doctor and practised medicine. He spent some time in psychiatry and developed private practice with people with mental health problems. Through his wide educational base, personal crises and his observation of patients, Freud developed a new and influential theory of the mind.

A key component of his theory was centred around the inner or unconscious conflicts that motivate a person's behaviour. However, he does suggest that some of these motivating conflicts (desires or thoughts) can become conscious through therapeutic techniques such as **free association, dream interpretation** and **transference**. Despite the contemporary significance of scientific development of knowledge and Freud's use of introspection and observation of patients, his psychodynamic theory has become part of everyday thoughts and the way of understanding the world.

Freud developed a structure of the mind, which is generally accepted by all psycho-dynamic theorists. The mind includes three components (see Figure 1.2):

- Id
- Ego
- Superego

Id

This is the part of personality or mind that a person is born with. It is the largest part of the unconscious structure of the mind. The **id** holds the sexual and aggressive instincts of the person and demands instant gratification. It is sometimes referred to as the 'psychic energy'.

Ego

This part of the personality or mind is the largest part of the conscious mind but at least half of it is **preconscious**. The **ego** develops in childhood and fulfils a function of balancing the desires of the id with the social constraints of the world which are internalised by the superego.

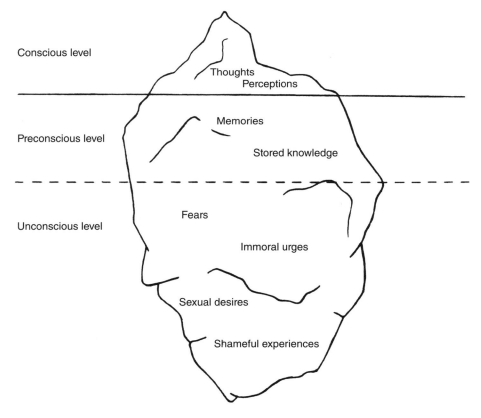

Figure 1.2   The psychodynamic mind represented as an iceberg

Superego

The **superego** is often referred to as the **conscience** of the person, which is considered to develop at about the age of five. The superego uses guilt and pride to persuade the ego to comply with social norms. The superego is partly conscious but also exists in the preconscious and unconscious.

Freud's theory also included a developmental process by which the structure of the mind and development of the personality were achieved. He suggested that children are born with the id but develop the ego and superego through psychosexual developmental stages. Freud identified that early childhood experiences go on to influence personality later in life (see Chapter 2 for theories on development).

Freud said that all behaviour is meaningful: no behaviour is accidental, whatever the behaviour. Any behaviour exhibited which the person's conscious mind had not intended is seen as unconscious thoughts breaking through to consciousness. These are generally referred to as 'Freudian slips'. Freudian slips, or **parapraxes**, are part of everyday language in Western societies. These Freudian slips are generally considered to have a sexual connotation: for example, the carer passes a cup of tea to a man she is caring for and he responds, 'Thank you for the *breast*s ... Tea, tea.' He had intended to say, 'Thank you for the *best* cup of tea,' but his noticing her breasts provoked him to say 'breast' instead of 'best'.

Activity 1.3   Reflection

Spend a few moments thinking of a time when you or someone else made a comment that made you feel embarrassed because it was not what you or they intended to say.

- Did it have a sexual interpretation?
- Can you identify what caused you or them to make the statement?

As this is a reflection, there is no outline answer at the end of the chapter.

Freud describes the mind as a dynamic structure in continuous conflict between the desires of the id and the social constraints of the superego. The ego's role is to resolve some of these conflicts and it will use mental defence mechanisms to achieve **equilibrium**. Mental defence mechanisms do not resolve anxieties or problems but allow the person to perceive them differently and manage their behaviour.

There is no agreed number of mental defence mechanisms; some suggest that there are just 9 and others propose 35. Nonetheless there is some agreement on their characteristics:

- They are unconscious, distinct and dynamic
- They can be adaptive or pathological
- They manage instincts, **drives** and feelings (Stewart, 2005)

In Table 1.2, you will find some examples of mental defence mechanisms, giving examples of how they may be seen in care practices.

Table 1.2   Freud's Mental Defence Mechanisms

Name of defence mechanism	Description	Example
Repression	Forcing a threatening memory/feeling/wish out of consciousness and making it unconscious	You feel sexually attracted to one of the people you are caring for but force this desire out of your consciousness
Displacement	Transferring feelings from their true target onto a harmless substitute target	One of the people you are caring for keeps calling you by the name of someone you do not like, but instead of reminding them of your name you go home and shout at your partner
Denial	Failing/refusing to acknowledge/perceive some aspect of **reality**	This can be observed when a family member refuses to acknowledge their loved one is dying
Rationalisation	Finding an acceptable excuse for some unacceptable behaviour	A person you have been supporting at great emotional expense makes a complaint about the amount of support they are receiving. You feel angry but say that this is due to their ill health
Reaction formation	Consciously feeling/thinking the opposite of your true (unconscious) feelings/thoughts	You strongly dislike a family member of a person you are caring for and so you become extremely considerate/polite towards them – even going out of your way to be nice to them
Sublimation	A form of displacement in which a substitute activity is found as a way of expressing some unacceptable impulse	You have been trying to encourage an older person to attend a hospital appointment. At the end of the shift, you feel very frustrated and so take yourself to the gym
Identification	Incorporating/introjecting another person into one's own personality – making them part of oneself	You are working with a woman who is being abused by her neighbour. When you suggest that she speaks to the police, she refuses as she says it is her own fault because she is demanding and stupid. The neighbour is working really hard and does a lot for her
Projection	Displacing your own unacceptable feelings/characteristics onto someone else	You find you are not able to relate to one of the people you are caring for and instead of saying that you do not get on with them, you say that they do not get on with you
Regression	Reverting to behaviour characteristic of an earlier stage of development	When asked to clean the kitchen for the second time that day, you lose your temper
Isolation	Separating contradictory thoughts/feelings into 'logic-tight' compartments	A person you have been caring for has taken their own life but you talk about it without any display of emotion

Source: Adapted from Barker (2007: 11)

In the case study of Miriam Walker, we can see that she may be using a number of mental defence mechanisms to facilitate compassionate care. Miriam may be **repressing** any irritation that she may feel at not being able to complete the paperwork; she may be **identifying** with Mr and Mrs Crosland's anxieties.

Summary

Freud offers a psychodynamic theory of the mind or personality and its development. He described mechanisms (mental defences) that a person might use to manage the continuous internal conflict of the different components within the mind. He steps beyond the dichotomy found in medicine and like Husserl identifies a mind that is embodied but also a distinct consciousness which has its own energy. This perspective offers care practitioners a different way to understand the people with whom they work and themselves. This will be further explored as the book progresses.

Behavioural psychology

Introduction

The behaviourists use scientific (experimental) methods to understand people's behaviour and behavioural change. Most of their theories have developed from animal experiments and models. They propose that all of a person's behaviour, including their personality (all individual differences), is learned. There are a number of processes by which this happens and they have become the building blocks of learning from a foundational level, called **habituation**, to more complex learning, called **social learning theory**.

Habituation

Habituation can be seen as the lowest form of learning on the hierarchy of learning. It is a process where the organism becomes 'used to' the presence of a stimulus, and is seen in the simplest of animals such as sea anemones. As with other types of learning, instead of habituation occurring, sensitivity can occur. For example, a person is sitting in a room with a ticking clock (Figure 3.1). After a little while, the person becomes 'used to', they habituate to, the noise of the clock and no longer notice it. For some, habituation does not occur and the person becomes more and more conscious of the ticking: they are **sensitised** to it.

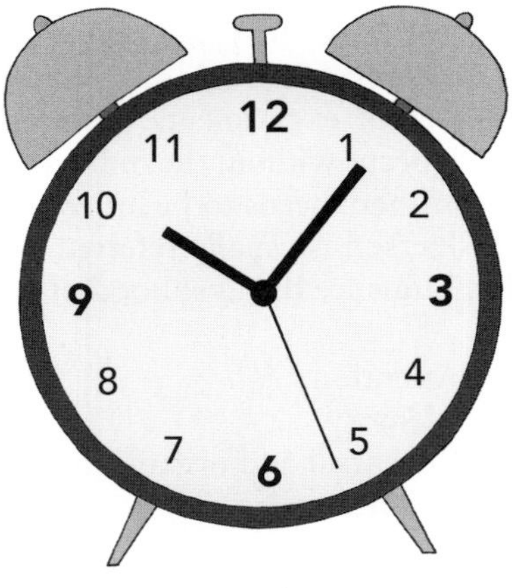

Figure 1.3   Clock

Classical conditioning

Classical conditioning is learning through **association**. This happens when one **stimulus** is presented with another and eventually they produce the same effect. This type of learning is usually considered **reflexive** learning, where the organism's reflex responses are being trained. The most famous experiment to demonstrate this was Pavlov's salivating dog study.

Ivan Pavlov (1849–1936) studied the digestive system of dogs. He recognised that dogs could be trained to salivate by pairing or associating another stimulus with food. Salivation is a reflex response to food. This **reflexive response** to food was **conditioned** to occur when a bell rang. The theory was later applied to people. It was found that pairing one stimulus with another stimulus could provoke a reflexive response in people. This is also called the **stimulus–response theory** of learning.

This has many applications in health and social care. For example, an older person with dementia has, from early learning, associated certain rituals with going to sleep.

They are then in the care environment facilitated to dress in their night clothes, the lights are turned down and the curtains closed (stimuli) so that they feel it is bedtime and fall asleep (response).

Operant conditioning

Learning can also occur by providing a reward or punishment when certain behaviour is enacted. This is called **operant conditioning**. This approach is widely used in schools, with animals and in society in general. For example, a child is given a star (**reward**) for their chart if they do something 'good' to encourage them to do it again but they have one removed (**punishment**) for 'bad' behaviour to stop it from happening again.

This type of learning was initially developed by Edward Thorndike (1874–1949), but Burrhus Frederic Skinner (1904–90) went on to extend this work. Skinner's empirical studies were, like Pavlov's, conducted on animals but subsequent studies have found that people also respond to classical and operant conditioning, although some people, as with habituation, respond in a way that is unexpected.

Social learning theory

Another form of learning that builds on the previous levels is more complex and higher on the hierarchy of learning. This is 'social learning theory'. This theory incorporates a cognitive element to learning. The theory accepts the previously established types of learning or conditioning but states that people, and we now find some other animals too, learn by observing others' behaviour and imitating it.

Albert Bandura and his colleagues developed this theory of social learning through a number of experiments. These demonstrated that observational or **vicarious** learning could occur without the individual being personally rewarded. For this type of learning to occur, there needs to be an appropriate environment with another person to learn from. This person is usually referred to as the **role model**. There are five cognitive components that influence the likelihood of learning from an environmental situation. These are:

- Attention
- Memory
- Rehearsal and organisation of memory
- Imitation
- Motivation

Activity 1.4   Critical thinking

Think of a person you admire and would like to be associated with; to be thought to be similar to. What did they do? Why do you want to do that?

An outline answer can be found at the end of the chapter.

Effective role models

There are features that are needed for a person to be an effective role model. They are:

- The role model is seen to be rewarded
- The role model is similar enough to the observer for them to imitate
- The role model is well thought of or respected in the social environment where the behaviour occurs

Returning to the case study of Miriam Walker, this perspective will indicate that she has learned to behave in certain ways. As a student, she will have been taught communication skills and observed her **mentor** (role model) assessing patients. She will have gained rewards (operant conditioning) by her mentor passing her on her necessary competencies and showing confidence in her ability by allowing her to speak to Mr and Mrs Crosland alone. By observing Mrs Crosland's behaviour, Miriam learned that asking her questions made her agitated and she did not get the answers. Miriam also learned from *observing* Mr Crosland's (role model) behaviour how to reduce agitation in Mrs Crosland; she *imitated* this and was able to make her assessment (social/vicarious learning).

The theories of behavioural psychologist have led to focused therapeutic approaches to health and well-being and these will be explored in Chapter 7.

Summary

There are four key types of learning identified by the behaviourists, although social learning theory does start to incorporate cognitive elements. Each of these theories is highly relevant to care practitioners for their personal development but also in developing the well-being of the people with whom they work. Proponents of all four types of learning accept that all behaviour is learned.

The four types of learning are:

- *Habituation*: The acknowledgement that people can 'get used to' or accept elements in their environment
- *Classical conditioning*: The training of reflexes such as pain by association
- *Operant conditioning*: If good things happen following certain behaviour, the person will repeat the behaviour
- *Social learning theory*: Care practitioners can learn from observing and imitating others

Cognitive psychology

Introduction

The cognitive perspective can be seen as a development of behaviourism because the early theorists came from behavioural psychology. They accept that behaviour is learned and that in any situation there is a stimulus and a response. It is based on the empirical scientific approach (see Chapter 5). Cognitive psychologists undertake experiments to determine how people process and structure their thoughts. They seek to understand what happens between stimulus and response because they recognise that not everyone responds in the same way to any given stimulus. This, in broad terms, is identified as cognition – conscious mental processing or thinking. Unlike Freud and the psychodynamic theorists, cognitive theorists do not concern themselves with the unconscious mind.

As the function of the mind and its precise link with the brain are not as clearly defined as it is with other organs in the body, it is difficult for psychologists to determine how and where information is stored and processing occurs. However, with the growth of technology and research in the area of bio- and neuropsychology, understanding is developing. Given the lack of biological models, cognitive psychologists tend to use metaphors, for example that the brain is an information processing unit like a computer. A computer goes through a logical system each time a problem is initiated. Some cognitive psychologists believe that people do the same thing, and they liken the brain to the hardware and the mind to the software.

Key influential areas in the development of the cognitive perspective are:

- Information theory
- Artificial intelligence (AI)
- Linguistics
- Neuroscience (Barker, 2007: 16)

Information processing approach

The 'information processing approach' is generally considered the major **paradigm** used in cognitive psychology to understand how people think. It is proposed that thinking is conducted in a logical, structured process. Cognitive psychologists have tried to map this process and structure. Components of this approach include:

- Set processing rules (organised ways in which information is gathered, stored, worked on and used)
- A storage facility for information (memory)
- A central processing unit which manipulates the information (a place where the information is worked on or with)

Schema theory

'Schema theory' is a cognitive theory of how people might store information and facilitate retrieval – memory. It is suggested that new information is attached to or becomes part of existing memory. A schema is a collection of information on a certain topic/area/thing. It has a **fixed component** but also has a **flexible component**. Schemas can be interrelated too, so that thinking about one schema can lead to a memory of information in another schema. For example, a 'giving an injection' schema, which may include dextral skills, syringes, needles, fluid to be injected, prescription, etc., may lead to a health and safety schema including objects like the sharps bin and skills such as washing hands (see Figure 1.4).

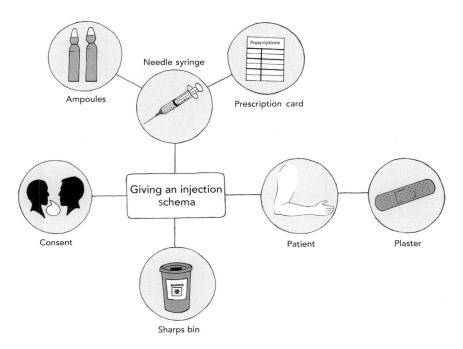

Figure 1.4 'Giving an injection' schema

Cognitive development theory

Jean Piaget (1896–1980) created a theory of cognitive development. Unlike the behaviourists, Piaget suggested that children of different ages think in a qualitatively different way to adults. His theory was built on a cognitive schema theory. He suggested that schemas were developed through a process of **assimilation** and **accommodation**.

- *Assimilation*: The process of incorporating new information into existing schemas
- *Accommodation*: Occurs when new information cannot be assimilated, at which point a new schema needs to be developed

Using this process, Piaget identified four stages of cognitive development: stage 1 also has six sub-stages. There have been a number of criticisms of Piaget's work but it continues to be influential, perhaps due to the scientific approach to its development of knowledge and understanding of the mind. This theory will be explored in more detail in Chapter 2.

The understanding of how people think is central within a number of therapeutic approaches to caring for them. These are explored in Chapter 7.

Summary

Cognitive psychologists offer a number of theories on how people think – they are particularly interested in cognitive processes and structures. These include the person's ability to communicate, attend and remember things. The information processing approach is the most common cognitive process approach, whereas the schema theory is the most widely accepted theory of how information is stored. Cognitive psychology offers an explanation for how people make decisions about their behaviour, including health and social behaviour. Clinical therapies have developed from cognitive psychology and these will be explored in Chapter 7.

Humanistic

Introduction

The humanistic movement is considered to have started in the 1950s as an alternative to the mechanistic and positivist approach taken by the behaviourists and the conflict and distress focused on by the psychodynamic psychologists. Whilst they accepted that learning (behaviourism) was important, they also acknowledged the importance of innate potential and unconscious processes (psychodynamic). Humanistic psychologists closely associated themselves with **existential** philosophy, with its roots in phenomenology. They were opposed to **positivism** and **rationalism**. They accepted that to understand the person we need recognise their existence, not focus on what comes directly to consciousness or that which can purely be observed. They suggest that people make decisions based on their subjective experiences, and not routinely in a rational, methodical manner. Each individual is therefore unique, as their world experiences are different (Barker, 2007).

Whilst humanist psychologists were influenced by philosophy, they developed individual theories to understand the person. Despite the theoretical differences and different focus in theoretical development, they all had a similar focus, which was optimistic. They identified that the person is an individual 'whole being' with their own unique **potential**. They also offered a spiritual element to psychological theory – there was something more in the experience than what could be measured or even labelled; they accepted psyche as mind and spirit. The humanists suggested that all people are moving towards **self-actualisation**: to achieve their potential. Whilst they believed that everyone was capable of achieving their own unique potential, they identified that unfavourable environments sometimes disrupt this journey (Rogers, 1961).

Alongside this focus, there are common themes within humanistic psychology. These are:

- Personal growth, potential, responsibility, self-direction
- Lifelong education
- Full emotional functioning
- Appreciation of joy and play
- Acceptance of **spirituality** and **altered states of consciousness** (Stewart, 2005)

Maslow

Abraham Maslow (1908–70) is generally considered the first humanistic psychologist; he developed the hierarchy of needs in 1954. He wrote that all people are motivated to fulfil their personal needs, and he organised these needs into a hierarchy which can be portrayed as a pyramid (Maslow, 1954) (Figure 1.5).

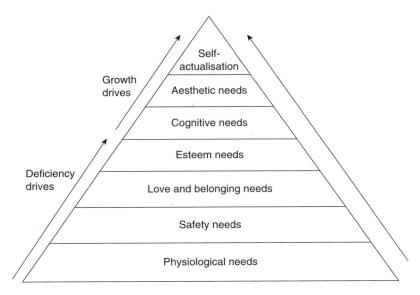

Figure 1.5 Maslow's (1954) hierarchy of needs

Maslow's hierarchy identified the order in which a person would fulfil their needs to achieve self-actualisation. He suggested that people have to work their way up from the bottom of the hierarchy to the top and they could not move to the next level until the needs of the previous one were fulfilled. The motivation to fulfil lower-level needs are identified as deficiency drives (4–7) which maintain health, and the motivation to fulfil higher-level needs are called 'growth drives' or 'being drives' (1–3). Both drives lead the person to self-actualisation, which can be visualised as a rapturous moment or peak experience:

1. Self-actualisation
2. Aesthetic needs
3. Cognitive needs
4. Esteem needs
5. Love and belonging needs
6. Safety needs
7. Physiological needs

Rogers

Carl Rogers (1902–87) developed what is now known as the person-centred approach which is advocated throughout health and social care. As with other humanists, he aligned himself with existential philosophy and regarded each person as unique. He stated that everyone is able to reach their own potential as long as they have the right environment in which they can grow towards self-actualisation.

Rogers developed a theory of self-concept which incorporated the actual self and the ideal self, and suggested that if these two views of the self were distant from each other a person would experience psychological distress – the person was **incongruent**. To gain a close ideal and actual self (**congruent** self), a person needs **unconditional positive regard**. Rogers went on to develop client-centred therapy to enable people who had not experienced this.

For effective client-centred therapy, Rogers identified a few necessary and sufficient elements:

- Two people need to be in psychological contact
- The client is in a state of incongruence
- The counsellor is congruent
- The counsellor experiences unconditional **positive regard** for the client
- The counsellor has an empathetic understanding of the client and endeavours to communicate this to the client
- The counsellor is at least successful in communicating unconditional positive regard and empathetic understanding to the client

Other theorists such as Gerard Egan have developed therapeutic interactions and interventions for people who need help based on the therapeutic and theoretical writing of Rogers. These will be further explored in other chapters of this book. It is accepted throughout this volume that to provide compassionate care there is a need to be person-centred, so this theory will be returned to in most chapters, particularly in Chapters 5 and 7.

If we return once again to Miriam Walker, we can clearly see that she is using humanistic approaches. She is showing *positive regard* to Mr and Mrs Crosland; they are in a state of *incongruence* and she is in a state of *congruence*; however, she did demonstrate a moment of incongruence when she became anxious as to whether Mrs Crosland had dementia. Miriam is facilitating their taking *responsibility* for their well-being by offering Mr Crosland the opportunity to fill in the forms and accepting their special relationship of understanding with each other (*spirituality/altered states of consciousness*).

Summary

The humanistic perspective is a collection of diverse theories but they have similar underlying principles. These principles are that:

- The person is motivated to self-actualise – they have the desire to achieve their potential
- The person is unique – each person is different
- The person has unique potential – each person has a different set of abilities, and they have an individual sense of fulfilment
- People need positive regard to remain healthy – to be acknowledged as having intrinsic value is important for well-being

Research methods in psychology

Introduction

There are a number of research methods used in psychology. Throughout this book, different philosophical approaches will be referred to and these influence what is considered credible or valid knowledge. Most psychologists tend to accept an empirical approach to gaining understanding and knowledge; *knowledge can only be gained through the senses or experiences*. Empirical knowledge is generally considered most credible globally but is usually viewed as scientific knowledge, achieved through the scientific process (see Chapter 5).

B.A. Carper in 1978 offered practitioners four ways of knowing, and identified empirical knowledge as only one way. The others were ethical knowing, aesthetical knowing and personal knowing. More recently, with the person-centred, compassionate care movement, other approaches to knowing are also being explored, such as intuitive knowing. As empirical knowledge is the most highly regarded, it will be considered first in this section of the chapter but other ways of knowing and understanding will be explored, as they are important if we are to ascertain how to become compassionate carers.

Empirical research

Empirical research studies are categorised into two groups: qualitative and quantitative research. Some, though, do not accept qualitative research as they focus on what 'comes to the senses', rather than the other part of empirical research of what 'is experienced' as well. They sometimes recognise qualitative approaches to be methods for facilitating ethical, personal and aesthetic ways of knowing, which are seen politically as less important. Most psychologists use the scientific approach in their search for knowledge but psychologists access research methods from a number of sources. Quantitative psychologists tend to adhere to the scientific method (used by biology, physics and chemistry), but qualitative researchers access methods from philosophy (phenomenology), sociology (grounded theory), anthropology (ethnography) and literary (narrative). It is only in the twenty-first century that qualitative research has become more accepted by psychology, with the British Psychological Society now having a section focused on this type of research.

Quantitative studies

Quantitative studies involve measuring an element of behaviour or behaviour change in a specific way: data would be collected so that it could be counted or measured. Most psychological research has been undertaken using this approach to understanding and it still has the greatest value politically. Methods include experiments, surveys and observations, but can include focus groups, diaries and interviews, where the literal data is converted into numerical data. This is the traditional scientific approach to research with a highly structured method. These studies are usually undertaken by biological, behavioural and cognitive psychologists.

Experiment and quasi-experimental methods

This quantitative method is used by positivists and accepted by the physical sciences to be valid as it has the ability to be rigorously tested. It uses the scientific procedure (see Chapter 5), and the findings are written up using the set scientific structure. This approach is where all unnecessary variables are eliminated from the experiment except those pertaining to the question or **hypothesis**. There are a number of experimental designs but the most valued is the **randomised control trial (RCT)**. The data gained is usually converted into numbers and made sense of by using **statistical analysis**.

Survey/questionnaire research

This method is used extensively to ascertain attitudes and other such social issues. The biological or cognitive psychologists and any psychologist interested in knowledge about behaviour in large populations may use this method. It is a method for gaining a small amount of information from a lot of people. As with the experimental approach, the data gained is usually converted into numbers and made sense of by using statistical analysis.

Observational research

This method is used extensively by behaviourists to assess stimulus–response situations: they observe for antecedents, behaviour and consequences. Biological and cognitive psychologists who may be observing for changes in behaviour may also use it. Piaget, who developed the cognitive development theory (see Chapter 2), used this approach to help develop his theory, along with experiments. The data in this research design again is usually converted into numbers and analysed statistically but the technique can also be used with small numbers of people.

Qualitative studies

Some psychologists do not recognise qualitative studies as empirical but they can, and some do, use the scientific approach, just exchanging the manipulated **variables** and hypotheses for research questions. These studies, though, seek narrative forms of data to maintain **ecological validity** and retain the richness of real-world experiences. They do not seek to measure or count behaviour. They usually include data collection through self-report diaries, reflections, interviews and focus groups. They are considered richer and seek to understand the human experience, and are more suited to the humanistic and psychodynamic perspectives.

Narrative

This approach to developing knowledge and understanding in psychology can be considered to have developed in literary, historical and social arenas. This is, though, too simplistic: the humanist's movement towards person-centred approaches and psychodynamic views of the person, along with structuralism, post-structuralism and postmodern philosophies, were also important (see Chapter 5). This approach seeks to gain **stories** of specific experiences, but given the diverse nature of its development and the many types of narrative approach, it might be considered an **umbrella** term. Generally, these different types of narrative research focus on the structure and form (**syntax**) of the language, and the **content** or the **genre** of the story. Psychologists from different perspectives may primarily use one type over another: for example, cognitive psychologists may be more interested in the form and structure of the story, whereas humanists may be more interested in the content, and psychodynamic psychologists in the genre, of the story.

Narrative research is about collecting stories and gaining understanding about the person or group of people by analysing the stories – the narratives.

Phenomenology

Phenomenology and existential philosophy have had a significant impact on the development of humanistic psychology (see Chapter 5). The philosopher Husserl is acknowledged as the founding father of phenomenology. He sought to find the essential experiences of a given phenomenon. Amedeo Giorgi, after studying Edmund Husserl and Maurice Merleau-Ponty, developed psychological phenomenology to provide researchers in psychology with a method to explore phenomena that maintained their unique character. Phenomenological research is usually conducted through lengthy in-depth individual interviews but can be undertaken by reading individual narrative descriptions of experiences of a phenomenon. It is important that the researcher maintains a state of **epoche** to elicit a description of **life world** experiences and to analyse these to elucidate the phenomenon using **imaginative variation**. The findings are usually presented as a **general structure** of the phenomenon along with **individual variations or constituents**. This research approach has been used by humanistic psychologists and psychotherapists, including those from a psychodynamic perspective.

Ethnography

This approach is used to describe and interpret cultural and social groups and has its origins in anthropology. Its focus is on describing and interpreting **cultural** groups: **culture-sharing groups**. Ethnographers explore learned patterns of behaviour, customs or ways of living. The researcher becomes involved in the culture and experiences it first-hand; they are **participant observers**. They make **field notes** and interview other people within the culture. They can also use **artefacts** – things produced by the culture. This data is then analysed and interpreted to develop cultural themes and develop a **cultural portrait**. This approach to research is of interest to social psychologists, whether they sit within behavioural, humanistic or psychodynamic psychological perspectives.

Grounded theory

Grounded theory developed from the discipline of sociology. As the name implies, this research approach aims to develop a theory of a particular situation from the **grounded** evidence, specific to the situation. The data is usually gained from interviewing people in the situation or **field**. Each interview is analysed and the next interview is conducted to build on the previously gained understanding. This is called a **constant comparative** method. The analysis is undertaken through different types of **coding** and **categorisation**. The researcher goes on to provide a theory or **storyline** that presents the central phenomenon and the social, historical and economic conditions that influence it. This research approach could be used by any of the psychological perspectives to explore different situations.

Psychologists can be seen to use every type of research approach available, and their choice of approach will depend on the perspective they align themselves with and what they are trying to understand about people. The perspectives, theories and research of psychologists will be used to explore our understanding of compassionate care and what it is, and how we can develop and maintain it in our caring relationships throughout the rest of this book.

Chapter summary

This chapter has taken us on a journey from the definitions of psychology, to an exploration of how psychology is organised and classified (perspectives), to psychologists' contemporary approaches to developing their knowledge (research).

Further study

The British Psychological Society website offers information on the different roles psychologists may take on. It offers guidance for those wishing to be a psychologist, as well as highlighting news, events and its publications. See: www.bps.org.uk/

Activity outline answers

Activity 1.1   Critical thinking

Take a few minutes to consider why an understanding of psychology might be useful in your development of your caring skills.
   You may have identified a number of ways in which it could be useful, such as:

- Helping you understand the person you are working with, your colleagues, your institution or company, your lecturers, yourself
- Helping you to identify how to help the person you are caring for, the awareness of therapeutic approaches, how to support and interact with others

Activity 1.4   Critical thinking

Think of a person you admire and would like to be associated with: to be thought to be similar to. What did they do? Why do you want to do that?

- Perhaps they managed to get someone to eat who was not eating, or to talk, walk or drink.
- Perhaps they received a smile or were able to undertake a technical or complex task.

Generally, our role models are displaying behaviour and being rewarded for doing something that we would like to achieve. Our role models also need to display behaviour that we feel we can imitate; if we do not feel we can imitate it (**self-efficacy**), we will not try.

References

Barker, S. (2007) *Vital Notes for Nurses: Psychology*. Oxford: Blackwell.
British Psychological Society (BPS) (2015) *Psychology*. Available at: www.bps.org.uk/ (accessed April 2015).
Carper, B.A. (1978) 'Fundamental patterns of knowing in nursing', *Advances in Nursing Science*, 1 (1): 13–24.
Ciccarelli, S.K. and Myer, G.E. (2006) *Psychology*. Upper Saddle River, NJ: Pearson Prentice Hall.
Colman, A.M. (2015) *A Dictionary of Psychology*, 4th edn. Oxford: Oxford University Press.
Maslow, A. (1954) *Motivation and Personality*. New York: Harper and Row.
Rogers, C.R. (1961) *A Therapist's View of Psychotherapy: On Becoming a Person*. London: Constable.
Stewart, W. (2005) *An A–Z of Counselling Theory and Practice*. Cheltenham: Nelson Thornes.

2 Lifespan Development

Sue Barker

Come, journey along life's road with me
A multitude of new experiences yet to be
Life's colourful tapestry ours to explore
Come, come change and grow old with me

Learning objectives

A psychological understanding of lifespan development is important for all care practitioners to provide compassionate care. This will support individual care needs as well as recognising the context in which people are growing and changing. This chapter's learning objectives are to:

- Discuss a variety of developmental theories and their psychological underpinning
- Explore how the knowledge of developmental theories can enhance the understanding of the group of people for whom compassionate care is shared

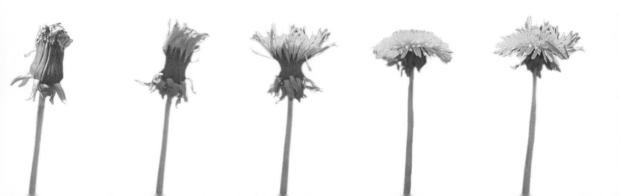

Introduction

This chapter will provide the philosophical background to the scientific understanding of development and lead to an exploration of the psychological theories of development. The psychological staged theories of development such as those of Piaget, Freud, Erik Erikson and John Bowlby will be focused on with a view to how these might inform caring practices.

> ## Activity 2.1   Critical thinking
>
> What do you think influences individual development? Do you think you are born to be the way you are or do you think your environment shaped you – the nature/nurture debate?
>
> *Some suggested answers can be found at the end of the chapter.*

Developmental theories

There are many developmental theories from various disciplines; for all of these, along with psychology, philosophical thought has provided a springboard for theory genesis (Table 2.1).

In the Middle Ages, it was assumed that people were preformed by God and just grew in size throughout their lifespan. The sperm was assumed to hold a very small person, a homunculus, which was inserted into the woman's womb and grew there until birth. This philosophy was known as 'preformationism', but to suggest that everyone thought this way is a bit simplistic because, during the sixteenth century, people such as King Henry VIII of England blamed his lack of a male heir on his wives. This would indicate the belief that women had some part in determining the sex of the baby.

The seventeenth century saw philosophical changes through what has been called the **Age of Enlightenment** or Age of Reason. This was where philosophers turned against accepting authority figures, such as the king or a priest, as the source of knowledge.

Table 2.1   Table of influential philosophers

Focus	Philosophers	Theorists	Psychological theorists	Further psychological theorists
Enlightenment/ Empiricists	Locke (1632–1704) Hume (1711–76)	Pavlov (1849–1936) Watson (1878–1958)	Skinner (1905–90)	Bandura (1925–)
Romanticists	Rousseau (1712–78)	Gesell (1880–1961)	Werner (1890–1964)	Piaget (1896–80)
Romanticists	Darwin (1809–82)	Lorenz (1903–89)	Bowlby (1907–90)	Ainsworth (1913–99)
Feelings/impulses	Brentano (1838–1917)	Freud (1856–1939)	Jung (1875–1961)	Erikson (1902–94)
Romanticists/ Phenomenologists/ Existentialists	Rousseau (1712–78) Kierkegaard (1813–55), Brentano (1838–1917)	Husserl (1859–1938) Heidegger (1844–1900)	Maslow (1908–70)	Rogers (1902–87)

It became accepted that knowledge was derived from reason and analysis and that people were individuals. John Locke (1632–1704), a philosopher at this time, influenced the behavioural or learning movement. The major theorists in this approach were Pavlov, Watson, Skinner and Bandura; all believed that the person starts as a *tabula rasa* (blank slate) – a term coined by Locke – and learns to be who they are through their environment.

Later, in the Age of Enlightenment, Jean-Jacques Rousseau (1712–78), a **Romantic Naturalist**, was to have a significant impact on developmental theories. Philosophers who are considered to be romanticists extol the virtues of nature and biological forces. He sparked the Romantic movement and initiated a psychological approach to development. Rousseau was a man of the Enlightenment and as such was willing to dismiss authoritarian ways of knowing and accept gaining knowledge by reason and analysis. Unlike the behaviourists, though, he was concerned with internally derived changes, in contrast to their external or environmental focus. He recognised that children are different to adults. They have their own modes of thinking, feeling and behaving and grow according to nature's plan.

Rousseau articulated four stages of development: stage 1, infancy (birth to 2); stage 2, childhood (2–12); stage 3, late childhood (12–15); and stage 4, adolescence (starts at puberty). This is called a **maturational theory** and many other theorists were to follow this approach such as Gesell, Werner and Piaget, but the evolutionary theories of Charles Darwin, Konrad Lorenz and Bowlby can also be seen to be influenced by Rousseau.

Arnold Gesell's (1880–1961) maturational theory followed Rousseau's belief that development occurs according to nature's plan. He adheres to two major factors affecting development: that people are a product of the environment and their genes. He stated that the sequence or order of development is fixed but rates or speed may vary. Gesell also said that anyone exploring development should consider patterns as well as quantitative concerns. At about the same time, Heinz Werner's (1890–1964), another follower of Rousseau, also saw the importance of patterns. Werner's maturational developmental theory was identified as **organismic** and **comparative**.

Werner saw development directed through the **orthogenetic principle**, where *ortho* means 'direction'; the principle is that genes ('genetic') provide the direction ('ortho') for development. It is a biological principle which establishes that development proceeds according to an internal plan. Werner's theory was organismic in that it viewed people as an integrated whole who have an inherent tendency to grow and develop. His theory was comparative as he suggested that development can be compared between different cultural groups of people. He argued that, whatever the culture, developmental achievements were comparable.

As with Gesell, Werner was interested in patterns such as those established by **gestalt philosophy**. He explored patterns of perception, cognition and language, accepting the orthogenetic principle, and identified development occurring through increasing **differentiation** and **hierarchic integration**. Differentiation is where parts of the person become distinct with their own functions and processes; for example, in the developing brain, structures develop that undertake specific tasks such as the visual cortex processing sight. Hierarchic integration occurs after differentiation facilitates separation of structures and their processes to hone their function more finely and incorporate them into an integrated whole body under its **hierarchical** management. For example, a baby watches its own hand and arm movement, the hand and arm are differentiated and the baby swings its arm in the air and clutches with its hand. The hand and arm

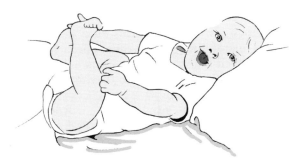

Figure 2.1 Baby moving its arms

are then hierarchically integrated – facilitating the baby's brain to control the finer movements of the hand and arm to fulfil the purpose of the baby (Figure 2.1).

Other post-Enlightenment philosophers who have influenced developmental theories in psychology are Brentano, Kierkegaard, Husserl and Heidegger. Brentano, discussed in more detail in Chapter 5, had a significant impact on both the psychodynamic theory of development as well as on the humanistic understanding of the person. Freud was a student at Brentano's school of philosophy at the same time as the philosopher Husserl, but their theories were to develop quite differently despite their joint understanding that the mind has psychic energy. Husserl's theory was to be labelled philosophical and Freud's psychological.

Heidegger was a student of Husserl and took over Husserl's academic post after he died. Whilst Heidegger was a phenomenologist, like Husserl, he also accepted the writings of Kierkegaard, the founder of the **existentialism** movement. Existentialism is an underlying philosophical approach accepted by the humanist movement and psychological humanistic theories such as Rogers' client-centred therapy.

As can clearly be seen, all psychological developmental theory has is origins in philosophical thought. The next section is going to explore the different psychological developmental theories.

Developmental psychology

Developmental psychology is the field of psychology which focuses on how people change and the ways in which they stay the same over a period of time. Developmental psychologists suggest that development is **systematic** and **adaptive** and occurs both **qualitatively** and **quantitatively** (Barker, 2007). Each psychological perspective offers a different way of understanding how people develop and change through their lifespan. Therefore, each psychological perspective will be considered in turn.

Biopsychologists

Biopsychologists accept a maturational theory of development based on biological changes that start prior to conception. There are many biological texts which will offer a detailed explanation of development from the early division of cells in the womb through to birth, childhood, puberty, childbirth, menopause, later life through to death. Biopsychologists, whilst accepting the maturational changes that occur throughout life due to these biological changes, are interested in how these impact on the person's feelings, behaviour and interactions with others.

Biopsychologists tend to focus on the brain and nervous system but look for **emergent properties**: things that cannot be predicted when studying an individual organ or structure. Another area of interest is where damage occurs and the person is unable to function in a manner expected. They explore the link between the biological structures and the **functional changes**.

As can be seen in the case study of Megan and Mollie, the biological structures of Mollie's brain did not develop as expected but this did not reduce the amount of love and compassion that could be shared between her and her family. Biopsychologists would be interested in how, despite the damage to Mollie's brain, she was still able to function well psychologically, personally and socially with others.

 ## Megan and Mollie Jones

Megan is the carer for Mollie and is also Mollie's mother. The birth had been a difficult one, with Megan traumatised; and Mollie had an **Apgar score** of four at birth but by five minutes this was seven. Mollie seemed to develop along the expected path until she reached one year old. Mollie was responsive to her mother and they had spent a lot of time smiling and making noises to each other. Both Megan and Mollie were very close and appeared happy in their relationship. Megan was not concerned when Mollie was not able to sit up independently until she was 10 months old as she was told babies develop at different rates. When Mollie was two years old, she was unable to speak more than a few words or to walk, and it was at this time that medical practitioners became concerned. Mollie had a brain scan: **magnetic resonance imaging (MRI)**. It was found that Mollie's brain was only 70 per cent of the weight of an adult brain and her cerebellum was significantly smaller. Mollie was a happy infant who smiled a lot and when sitting in her 'buggy' no one thought she was different from any other little girl. Mollie did not seem frustrated by her inability to keep up with her younger sister, who she enjoyed watching. Megan, whilst being concerned for Mollie, felt that Mollie brought her and the whole family great happiness.

Case study

Behaviourists

The Behaviourist movement was built on the empirical philosophy of Locke and Hume. They were to influence the research of Pavlov, Watson and Skinner. It was established by them that only what comes to the senses can be considered real or truth. They accepted that when a child is born, it is a 'blank slate' with the ability to learn but with no innate knowledge of themselves or others. As the child grows, it learns who it is and how to behave through its environment. They did not distinguish between the innate skills of people and other animals and therefore accepted the application of animal models to human experience.

The behaviourists accept that people throughout their lifespan develop using the same methods in their endeavour to behave in the most rewarding way. These methods of learning were outlined in Chapter 1 but include habituation, classical conditioning, operant conditioning and vicarious learning (social learning). Behaviourists are not interested in any other type of development as they believe that only what can be assessed through the senses, observed or measured, in some manner, has any validity so they measure and observe behaviour. Whilst this may appear to be a limited view of human development, it has led to a number of very helpful therapeutic approaches, which will be explored in Chapter 7 of this book.

Case study

Janet Lowe – a nursery nurse

A mother approached me and appeared quite distressed by her 3-year-old son's behaviour. She had found him prodding his baby sister with a sharp pencil when she was lying asleep in the sitting room. She said she thought that he was jealous and trying to harm his sister. I explained to the mother that I could see why this would upset her but suggested there may be other reasons for his behaviour. We discussed how we could check out why he was behaving this way and agreed to fill in an antecedent, behaviour and consequence (ABC) template each time it happened. The mother was more vigilant than usual and filled in the template in detail. The little boy was found to prod his sister with a pencil through a gap between the hood and the seat when she was in her 'buggy'. He usually did this when she was having her afternoon 'nap' in the sitting room. He did not do it immediately after the mother left the room – it was usually about five minutes after she had left. When the mother caught him doing this, she raised her voice and told him it was very naughty and he cried.

I also asked the mother to complete a diary of what she did when she was in the room whilst her daughter was asleep. The mother was surprised to find that every 5 to 10 minutes she would walk over to the 'buggy', look at her daughter, gently stroke her face and then return to her seat.

I did not need to offer the mother an alternative explanation for her son's behaviour as she was able to recognise that his behaviour was mirroring hers in the only way available to him. After this point, instead of trying to protect her daughter from an aggressive and jealous brother, she put her daughter on a quilt on the floor for her afternoon sleep. She found that her son now, if left for a few minutes, went over to his sister and softly stroked her face. She then approached him and said what a good boy he was and gave him a hug.

In the scenario shared by Janet, we can see that the little boy was developing an understanding of how to behave by watching his mother. He could not follow all her behaviour as he was too small, but he had learned that he could use a pencil to touch his sister. His sister waking up and crying may have been a **reinforcement** of this behaviour as his mother returned to the room and took over 'care' for his sister.

There could be a number of internal processes involved in his choice of behaviour, but according to the behaviourists he and his mother will not be able to determine what these are at the moment as only the overt behaviour is available to the senses. The mother's behaviour when he stroked his sister's face could offer a reward to the boy, and he will learn through operant conditioning that this is a 'good'/rewarding way to behave.

The behaviourist view of people developing by using their innate ability to learn can clearly be seen in the case study presented by Janet.

Psychodynamic approach to development

As outlined in Chapter 1, Freud was the founder of the psychodynamic perspective and has been influenced by the philosophical approach of the Enlightenment, **empiricism** and Brentano. There are also many similarities to the maturational theory of Rousseau in his psychosexual developmental theory. This is not surprising as Freud was a man of his time and, given the developing biological understanding of the body, he gained through his education in medical science. The medical sciences would not have achieved the contemporary understanding of the human without the philosophical underpinning of the Enlightenment, empiricism and romanticism.

However, Freud's education included spending some time at Brentano's school, where he recognised that there was more to the person than biological structures and processes. Along with Husserl, he claimed that humans had an additional psychic energy. Freud initially called this the individual's **libido** or life force. Later in his life, he was to describe the forces of **Eros** and **Thanos**, too: the motivation to live (Eros) and to die (Thanos). This life force provides the energy for the person to move through a maturational process to become themselves – to achieve a full **self-concept**. Freud's model of the personality is outlined in Chapter 1; it involves an unconscious part (the largest part, mostly made up of the id but also containing superego and ego), preconscious part (the next largest part, mostly the ego) and conscious part (the smallest part, ego and superego).

It is Freud's maturational process that will be explored in this part of this chapter. Freud described the child as undergoing five psychosexual stages, the timings of which can be seen as being very similar to those of Rousseau. Freud's focus was on how, through interaction with the world motivated by the libido, infants' and children's relationships with themselves and others changed.

The five psychosexual stages described by Freud are:

- Oral stage (0–2 years)
- Anal stage (2–4 years)
- Phallic stage (4 to middle childhood)
- Latency stage (middle childhood)
- Genital stage (adolescence through to adulthood)

Freud indicated that each stage needed to be completed at the appropriate maturational moment and that if a child was over- or under-stimulated at any stage, then they may become **fixated** at that stage and this would limit their adult personality. They may also return to a fixated stage at times of adult stress (**regression**) or develop an ongoing personality type linked to that stage.

Oral stage (0–2 years)

Any observation of a young infant will demonstrate that the focus at this time is around the mouth: oral. The infant is mainly interested in seeking food, exploring the world and stimulation using its mouth: new objects will be explored orally. Therefore, if an adult is fixated or regresses to this stage, they are likely to display activities related to their mouth. This may be seen in excessive eating or by dieting and binge eating, drinking to excess or smoking. Two sub-stages have been identified as:

- *Oral eroticism*: This is where sucking and eating are dominant behaviours and people with an oral erotic personality are likely to be cheerful but dependent and needy
- *Oral sadism*: For these people, biting and chewing predominate and the person is said to exhibit cynicism and cruelty (Barker, 2007: 34)

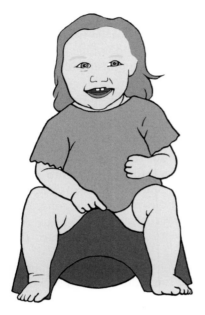

Figure 2.2 Toddler on a potty

Anal stage (2–4 years)

For an average child during the second to fifth year, prior to attending school, they are likely to be going through a period of toilet training (Figure 2.2). Early in this stage they are also developing some sense of autonomy, which is usually called the 'terrible twos'. This sense of autonomy may be linked to the child's recognition that they may have some control over their body through their choosing when to urinate or defecate. The child may also become fascinated with not only their own ability but other people's ability to control their elimination. With the anal stage two sub-stages or personality types have also been identified:

- *Anal-retentive*: This sub-stage is said to involve the desire to hold on to waste products; people that regress to this stage or are fixated here are considered to be excessively neat, clean, meticulous and obsessive
- *Anal-expulsive*: People in this sub-stage considered to be moody, sarcastic, biting and often aggressive. Retentive and expulsive are defined as opposites, but a person can move from one to another depending on circumstances (Barker, 2007: 35).

Phallic stage (4 to middle childhood)

For Freud, this stage was seen to be pivotal in the child's development, and he spent a lot of energy thinking and writing about this stage. This is the stage where the child struggles with the **oedipal** complex, sometimes called the **electra** complex in females. Children start to recognise their sexual identities and through relationships with their parents set the foundations for future sexual relationships. For Freud, if gender identity is not achieved at this stage the child may go on to find itself attracted to same-sex partners. People who regress to or are fixated in this stage are said to be overly preoccupied with themselves; they are considered to be **narcissistic**. They are said to be vain and arrogant and exude an unrealistic level of self-confidence, as well as self-absorption.

Activity 2.2   Reflection

In Freud's theory, successfully working through the oedipal and electra complexes leads to girls finding men who are more similar to their fathers more attractive than other men, and likewise boys are attracted to women like their mothers. Think about the people you find sexually attractive. Do your attractions comply with Freud's theory?

As this is a reflection, there is no outline answer at the end of the chapter.

Latency stage (middle childhood)

This is a quiet stage of development according to Freud's psychosexual development. People fixated or regressing to this developmental stage demonstrate sexual **sublimation** and repression of sexual desires (mental defence mechanisms; see Chapter 1 for more detail).

Genital stage (adolescence through to adulthood)

This is the final stage of psychosexual development according to Freud, and if the person has not fixated at an earlier stage they should achieve normal adult sexuality and a full self-concept at this time, as defined by Freud (i.e. traditional sex roles and heterosexual orientation).

Erikson's theory of psychosocial development

Erik Erikson (1902–94) was also a psychodynamic theorist and accepted the structure of the mind developed by Freud, but Erikson suggested that development continued throughout the lifespan. He based this on anthropological studies. He proposed eight stages from the beginning of life to the end of the lifespan (Table 2.2). The stages are **polar**, with a negative and a positive polar extreme. Each stage is described as a **crisis**: a time of change. For successful achievement of the stage the developing person needs to achieve a balance between the opposing polarity. If a balance is achieved the person will gain a **virtue** or **ego strength**. Erikson accepted that stages could be revisited but this would be problematic for the developing person.

Stage 1: Basic trust versus mistrust

Stage 1 lasts from the child's birth to 12–18 months old, and at this time the baby develops a sense of whether the world is a good and safe place. The theory suggests that a balance between trust and mistrust is important. If a child completely trusts everyone and everything in the world then it will put itself in danger, but if a child mistrusts the world it will live in continuous fear. Therefore, a child needs to feel safe and secure but also to recognise that there are dangers in the world.

If the balance is achieved, the ego strength or virtue of HOPE is gained.

Table 2.2   Erikson's psychosocial developmental theory

Stage	Poles	Age	Virtue/ego strength
1.	Trust versus mistrust	0 to 12–18 months	Hope
2.	Autonomy versus shame	12–18 months to 3 years	Will
3.	Initiative versus guilt	3–6 years	Purpose
4.	Industry versus inferiority	6 to puberty	Skill
5.	Identity versus identity confusion	Adolescence to young adult	Fidelity
6.	Intimacy versus isolation	Young adulthood	Love
7.	Generativity versus stagnation	Middle adulthood	Care
8.	Integrity versus despair	Older adulthood	Wisdom

Stage 2: Autonomy versus shame

In Stage 2, the child is 12–18 months to 3 years old and working through the crisis of independence versus shame and doubt. Children are learning the language of their culture and developing skills such as control over their elimination. It is a time when the child is starting to take control over its body and feel some responsibility for its behaviour. If the child manages this well they gain autonomy, but if this becomes a problem for them they may experience shame. The search for autonomy can lead them into conflict with adults, and this time is frequently called the 'terrible twos'. Again, a balance is needed so that the child gains some autonomy and a sense of responsibility which can lead to shame.

If the balance is achieved, the virtue of WILL is gained.

Stage 3: Initiative versus guilt

This stage is similar to the previous one as the child of 3–6 years old is having lots of new experiences and developing its autonomy and sense of self through using its initiative. The child has competing desires: it desires to achieve new things and be competitive (to use its initiative), but it also desires to be approved of by others, especially by its family (which may lead to guilt). The child needs to balance its desires so that it can gain achievements but within the social boundaries.

If the balance is achieved, the virtue of PURPOSE is gained.

Stage 4: Industry/competence versus inferiority

The ages of this stage are less well defined than the previous stages as it depends on the start of puberty, which varies according to the availability of food, infection rates and differences between cultures (Pierce and Hardy, 2012). In Western societies, where puberty in girls was seen to start at approximately 13 years of age in the 1970s, the age of puberty is decreasing, with approximately 30 per cent of girls in the USA achieving puberty at 8 (Biro et al., 2010).

The child starts this stage at approximately 6 years old and completes it at puberty. It is a time for the learning skills (industry) of the culture or facing feelings of incompetence (inferiority). If the child assesses themselves to be competent/industrious they may achieve high self-esteem. As with previous crises, the child needs to gain a balance so that it is not over-confident and is able to maintain its social relationship as well as recognising its skills.

If a balance is achieved, the child will gain the virtue of SKILL.

Stage 5: Identity versus identity/role confusion

This stage is called 'adolescence' and covers the period from puberty to young adulthood. The adolescent at this stage is exploring who they are and what their role in society is. According to Erikson, this sense of self allows the person to develop intimate relationships in the next stage, to plan for the future, to focus on their goals such as their career and to reduce risk-taking behaviours. However, Erikson identified that for women, stages 5 and 6 may be reversed. Women may find a sense of self through their intimate relationships with others.

If achieved, the young person will gain the virtue or ego strength of FIDELITY.

Stage 6: Intimacy versus isolation

Stage 6 is one of young adulthood: at this time, the person seeks to make commitments to others and develop close intimate relationships to avoid isolation. During this stage, the young person tries to hold onto their sense of self at the same time as becoming part of someone else (Figure 2.3). They develop a sense of duty and responsibility to and for the other person. If the person successfully achieves this stage, they may gain a loving relationship whilst still knowing themselves and having a robust self-concept. If the person is unsuccessful, they may suffer from isolation and self-absorption.

If achieved, the person will gain the virtue or ego strength of LOVE.

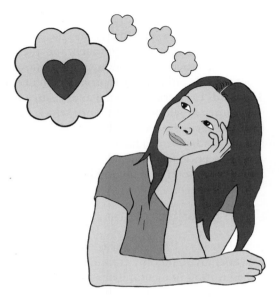

Figure 2.3   Woman in love

Stage 7: Generativity versus stagnation

Middle adulthood involves a crisis that is frequently labelled the 'midlife crisis'. In Stage 7, the mature adult's focus is on developing and guiding their families, local communities and the next generation. These adults need to feel that they are achieving something that is meaningful and that will enhance the well-being of others. If they are unable to do this, they can be left with a feeling of personal impoverishment and will become preoccupied with their own needs.

If achieved, the person will gain the virtue or ego strength of CARE.

Stage 8: Integrity versus despair

This is the stage of late adulthood and, similar to puberty, its timing is very different from the context of when Erikson developed his theory in the 1960s and 1970s. In the 1960s, men in the UK could expect to live to 68 and women had a life expectancy of 73 (Willets et al., 2004). Life expectancy has increased, with average life expectancy rising to approximately 79 years for men and 83 for women in the UK (ONS, 2014). For Erikson, late adulthood is where older people need to achieve acceptance of their own life and acceptance of the inevitability of death. This involves acknowledging the things that have not gone the way they hoped but also accepting what they have achieved. It is a coming-to-terms with their personal imperfections of their own humanity and **celebrating** who they are. It is also accepting and coming to terms with the imperfections of others including their parents. He states that if the older person is unable to achieve this, they may experience despair over their inability to relive life, to improve what has not gone well (Barker, 2007).

A successful completion of this crisis leads to the virtue or strength of WISDOM.

Whilst Erikson's theory may be believed to be 'of its time', particularly with the widening of the period between puberty and the end of life, his theory was the first to offer a whole lifespan developmental approach and there is still much to be learned from it. It has encouraged social and healthcare practitioners to see older people as still having developmental needs rather than approaching older age as a time of reduction and entrenchment. This leads to restricting social and leisure contacts and a focusing on physical care needs.

Another developmental theory which focuses on the early years of life from the psychodynamic perspective is Bowlby's theory of attachment. Whilst Erikson's psychosocial theory can be seen to have been influential in the development of thinking and research in adolescence, mid-life and older people, Bowlby's research and theory has been pivotal in the provision of social and healthcare for children.

John Bowlby's theory of attachment

John Bowlby (1907–90) was employed as a child psychiatrist and in this role used his psychoanalytic therapy training. Most psychiatrists after their medical training and initial education in mental illnesses still access developmental opportunities within psychological therapies. Through his work with young people who had mental health problems and offending behaviours, Bowlby became interested in **attachment**. He explored the research of Konrad Lorenz, an **ethologist** (a person who studies animal behaviour). Lorenz's research focused on **bonding** and **imprinting**. He was particularly famous for his work with geese, and he identified that for certain animals there was a critical time in which they bonded or imprinted onto their mother. His work with geese demonstrated that it was the critical time that was significant, not the presence of the mother, as his geese imprinted on other inanimate objects in his experiments (Figure 2.4).

Ethologists like Lorenz, through their animal studies, originally defined attachment as early imprinting or bonding, but Bowlby's work became the defining theory of human attachment. Between 1950 and 1988, Bowlby developed and refined the concept of attachment. He defined attachment as an intimate, warm, continuous relationship between mother and baby where both find satisfaction and enjoyment (Bowlby, 1951).

Bowlby, by studying the writings of Lorenz and Freud alongside his clinical work and research, proposed a critical period for attachment in people of between six months and 3 years of age (stage 1 for Rousseau's and stage 1 and part of stage 2 for Freud's and Erikson's theories). Bowlby stated that at this time the infant needs continuous love and care from

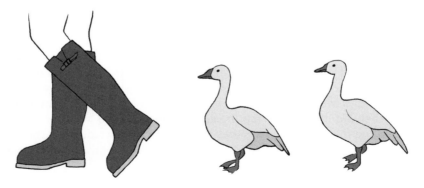

Figure 2.4 Geese following wellies

one person, the mother or mother substitute. Significant separations during this period would have a serious negative impact on the emotional and social development of the child.

Bowlby (1951) said that attachment with their mother is as important for the baby's mental health as nutrition is for physical health. He proposed the concept of **monotropy,** which identifies that the baby's attachment to their mother is qualitatively different from any other later attachments. He clearly stated that without this attachment children could become **affectionless psychopaths.**

Bowlby went on to develop a model of how this lack of early attachment might have long-term effects on the person. He called this model the **internal working model** (see Figure 2.5).

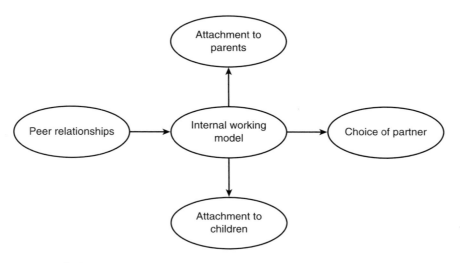

Figure 2.5 Bowlby's internal working model

Bowlby stated that early life experiences lead the infant to develop certain beliefs and expectations about the world and their relationships. If the infant has received continuous love from its mother then it will develop the belief that people can be trusted, that they are, personally, worthy of love and that people care. This is a similar position to Erikson's, but Erikson did not identify that the trust needed to be developed through a relationship between baby and mother. Bowlby believed that this early relationship with the mother would form the pattern for future relationships including those with their own children. A strong trusting relationship with the mother allowed the child to develop the expectation that the world is a benevolent place, which can be **self-reinforcing** – a **self-fulfilling prophecy.**

Mary Ainsworth was a student of Bowlby and developed his research on attachment. She, along with her assistant Barbara Wittig (Ainsworth and Wittig, 1969), developed a technique to assess whether infants were attached to their mothers. This became known as **the strange situation.** Using this technique, Ainsworth and her colleagues (Ainsworth et al., 1976) found three types of attachment:

- *Type A*: Anxious – avoidant
- *Type B*: Securely attached
- *Type C*: Anxious – resistant

These different types of attachment have been found to affect not only the child's behaviour but also their behaviour as adults, as predicted by Bowlby's internal working model.

Bowlby used the term **deprivation** to label what occurs when a child has problems with attachment to their mother. This was later divided into deprivation and **privation**. Privation is defined as when there has been no opportunity for the child to develop an attachment, for example children in institutionalised care. Deprivation is less severe and occurs when the child has developed an attachment but experienced an element of separation or loss in the relationship. These two terms are believed to have different outcomes for the child.

Activity 2.3   Critical thinking

Bowlby said that only 60 per cent of mothers develop secure attachments with their children. What are the implications for society and care practitioners?

There is an outline answer at the end of the chapter.

The impact of deprivation depends on the longevity of the disruption: short-term disruption can lead to distress (protest, despair, detachment), but in long-term separation this can lead to anxiety (aggression, clinging, detachment or physical health problems). Privation is more severe and a longer-term problem which could lead to developmental problems or, using Bowlby's term, 'affectionless psychopathy'. As indicated at the beginning of this section, Bowlby's research has been influential in further research and been used in the development of health and social care services.

One influential piece of research it stimulated was undertaken by James and Joyce Robertson from 1967 to 73. They recorded a series of short silent films in black and white which had a dramatic impact on hospital practice in the care of children. These powerful films demonstrated the emotional impact on children of deprivation of their mothers. The screening of these films led to children and parents having open access to each other in hospital settings and more community-based care for children.

Psychodynamically underpinned theories of development emphasise the importance of achieving psychological developmental milestones, particularly those in the early years of life, not only for a psychologically healthy childhood but also to offer a secure base for adult life.

Cognitive approach to development

The cognitive perspective grew out of behaviourism when it was recognised that a pure stimulus response mechanism was inadequate for predicting humans' behaviour. As with the psychodynamic approach but unlike behaviourism, this perspective offers a staged theory of development. Cognitive theorists, including those interested in development, such as Piaget, are concerned with changes in mental abilities such as learning, memory, **reasoning**, thinking and language.

Piaget's cognitive theory of development

In the 1930s, Piaget suggested that children think in a qualitatively different way to adults, rather than just having less knowledge – following the philosophy of Rousseau and the romantics. His theory outlined how cognitive development progressed through the interaction of innate capabilities (romanticism) with environmental events (empiricism) through four distinct hierarchical stages. His theory is very similar to Werner's developmental theory. Piaget's theory is a maturational theory, which utilises the cognitive concept of **schemas**.

Schema theory

A schema is explained as the building block of intelligent behaviour. Schemas are mental structures which provide a mechanism to organise past experiences and to understand new ones. Schemas or pockets of knowledge are developed, according to Piaget, through a process of assimilation and accommodation in order to achieve equilibrium (see Figure 1.4).

Assimilation

Assimilation is the bringing-together of new information into an existing schema: a group of thoughts, memories, experiences related to a specific thing (such as a dog, riding, love).

For example, you may have a schema for a person with dementia. Your schema is that people with dementia are old, unable to speak or dress themselves and cannot remember who they or their family are. You visit a friend whose father has dementia; when you arrive at the door you are welcomed by a smart but casually dressed man who smiles and invites you into the house saying you must be his daughter's friend. You feel uncomfortable because either your friend has misinformed you as this man does not 'fit' with your schema of a person with dementia, or this is not her father. Due to this experience of **cognitive dissonance**, you need to adapt your schema to feel more comfortable, to return to equilibrium or **homeostasis**.

Activity 2.4   Critical thinking

Schema theory suggests that cognitive dissonance causes a person to reorganise their schema or stereotype of a person/incident/object, etc. How might you experience cognitive dissonance?

There is an outline answer at the end of the chapter.

Accommodation

Accommodation occurs when new information cannot be assimilated into an existing schema. Accommodation induces the old schema to be changed or a new one to be developed. It is where an existing schema needs to be changed or a new one to be developed so as to include new information.

Returning to the example of meeting a person with dementia above: your friend's father invites you to sit down and says that his daughter has just gone to the shop but will be back in a few minutes. He asks you if you would like a drink as he is about to have a coffee; you agree to join him in having a coffee. He proficiently proceeds to make a cafetière of coffee, laying up a tray with cups, milk, sugar and biscuits. Whilst doing this, he tells you an amusing story about why his daughter needed to go to the shops.

At this point, your cognitive dissonance increases as you are unable to incorporate this experience into your previously held schema. To regain cognitive equilibrium, you develop a new schema about people with dementia.

As previously stated, Piaget, along with Rousseau, identified that infants and children think in a qualitatively different way to adults and both offered a staged theory of development. Piaget identified four stages of development which used the processes of assimilation and accommodation for the child to progress to adult thinking patterns (Table 2.3).

Table 2.3   Piaget's cognitive developmental stages

Stage	Age group	Major achievements
Sensorimotor stage	0–2 years old	Object permanence
Preoperational stage	2–7 years old	Symbolic representation, classification, cause and effect, **number concepts**
Concrete operations	7–11 years old	Conservation, serialise, distinguish fact from fantasy
Formal operations	11 years onwards	Hypothetical deductive reasoning

Piaget's four stages of cognitive development

Sensorimotor stage: 0–2 years old

During this stage, the newly born infant progresses from total dependency to independent mobility and social interaction. Cognitively, the baby has developed physical schemas to control its bodily movements and a sense of **object permanence**. See Table 2.4 for details on the sub-stages of this stage.

Table 2.4   The sub-stages of Piaget's sensorimotor stage

Sub-stage	Age	Skills
1. Reflexive activity	Birth to 1 month	Activities or physical schemas used are reflexive. Infants are refining their **innate** responses, e.g. sucking
2. Primary circular reactions	1–4 months	Actions which happen by chance are repeated when behaviour is rewarded, e.g. moving thumb to mouth to suck it. No sense of object permanence
3. Secondary circular reactions	4–8 months	The infant uses established schemas to explore new objects, e.g. the baby will suck a new toy which it is given

Sub-stage	Age	Skills
4. Coordination of secondary schemas	8–12 months	Child coordinates previously learned schemas and is able to use learned behaviour to achieve goals, e.g. the baby will push things out of the way to get to a toy. At this stage, it has some sense of object permanence
5. Tertiary circular reactions	12–18 months	Child uses trial-and-error strategies to achieve goals and experiment with objects, e.g. dropping them out of their pushchair and then looking for them
6. New means through mental combinations	18–24 months	Symbolic activity starts to appear and a child can use a sound or action to represent an object not there, e.g. making the noise and action of an aeroplane. They show signs of problem-solving and have a sense of object permanence

Source: Adapted from Davey (2004: 301)

Preoperational stage: 2–7 years old

At this stage, the child has had some qualitatively different thinking achievements from the previous stage, but there are still many limitations to cognitive ability (see Table 2.5).

Table 2.5 Preoperational stage achievements and limitations

Achievements	Limitations
Uses representational systems (i.e. words)	**Centration** – inability to decentre: the child can only focus on one element at a time
Understanding of cause and effect (why things happen)	**Conservation** – number, length, liquid, matter, weight, area; the child does not recognise that they will stay the same if the local environment changes
Ability to classify (e.g. all brown together)	Inability to distinguish appearance from reality
Understanding of number concepts • **1-to-1 principle** (each item has one number) • **stable-order principle** (numbers always go in a set order: 1, 2, 3 ...) • **order-irrelevance principle** (it does not matter where you start, you still have the same number of the given items) • **cardinality principle** (the last number said when counting is the number of items) • **abstraction principle** (counting can be applied to many things)	**Irreversibility** – unable to see that an action can go both ways **Transductive reasoning** – sees cause where none exists **Egocentrism** – assumes that everyone thinks as they do **Animism** – attributes life to inanimate objects

Midwife Annie Davies

I was visiting a newly delivered mother at her home, and her five-year-old daughter Maisie was observing my examination. After a while, Masie asked me: 'Are you going to come every day?' I explained that I would be visiting for the next five days and showed her the days on the calendar. The child happily counted the days (demonstrating the **stable-order principle**), starting with the first day I showed her and then she started again with the last day and both times reached the conclusion I was going to visit for five days (*order-irrelevance principle*). Maisie then asked: 'Is your mother going to be sad you being with us?' (*egocentrism and centration*). I explained that I will come to visit them for an hour each day and then go home again. Maisie then looked confused and said: 'But how can you go home again?' (*irreversibility*). I explained that I will go home in my car and showed Maisie my car out of the window. She then brightly exclaimed, as if finally understanding, that I could not stay with them because my car would be sad (*animism and transductive reasoning*) but that I would come back in five days.

The next stage finds the child achieving the limitations of this stage.

Concrete operations stage: 7–11 years old

When a child reaches the concrete operational stage, they are able to achieve thinking that had not been available to them at the preoperational stage. They have the ability to:

- Conserve/classify (**classification**) – class inclusion (an object can be in more than one class)
- **Serialise** – e.g. organisation of darkest to lightest
- Distinguish between fantasy and reality
- Understand **cause and effect** – each time one thing happens, another thing happens because of it

Formal operations: 11 years onwards

At this stage, the child develops adult thinking processes which facilitate their imaginative and abstract thinking. They develop the ability to use **hypothetical deductive reasoning** (working things out step by step in their head) and can manipulate ideas or propositions. However, it is suggested that many children never achieve this level of cognition.

Humanistic approach to development

This perspective was developed in response to the empirical behaviourists and the romanticism of Freud. Whilst the humanists accepted many of these philosophies and psychological theories, they found them lacking in some essential elements to offer a true representation of people. Humanistic theorists built on previous psychological theories and on the philosophies of empiricism, romanticism, phenomenology and existentialism.

As stated in the previous chapter, humanistic psychology has these themes in common:

- Personal growth, potential, responsibility, self-direction
- Lifelong education
- Full emotional functioning
- Appreciation of joy and play
- Acceptance of spirituality and altered states of consciousness (Stewart, 2013: 230)

Unlike biopsychologists, psychodynamic or cognitive psychologists, humanistic psychologists do not offer a staged theory of development. They do, however, state the environmental needs for a person to reach their potential, and in this case they can be seen to be similar to the behaviourists. They also accept an innate energy or motivational force identified by Freud and psychodynamic theorists.

People, humans, can reach their potential or self-actualisation at any point in their life's journey but as they develop and grow, their unique potential will grow as well. Therefore, there will always be more room for development and change. To maintain personal growth, full emotional functioning, appreciation of joy and an acceptance of their spirituality, the person needs to be continually moving towards their potential and self-actualisation.

This is achieved by fulfilling their growth and deficiency needs (Maslow) within an environment where the person is acknowledged and respected (Rogers). The person is always in a state of becoming (Stewart, 2013), and receiving positive regard enables the person to give positive regard to others.

 ## Daisy Dillon – mental health nurse

Case study

I have worked with a number of young women with a diagnosis of personality disorder, but one I remember more than the others because, as I moved from inpatient working to the community, Sharon moved with me. I found Sharon really difficult and I was not very happy about her 'following' me but I think we grew together over time. Whilst an inpatient, Sharon was doing all the things that the staff found difficult; she idolised some staff – not me – and others she bedevilled. As soon as we thought she was doing well, she would self-harm by cutting herself. Everyone wanted her off the unit, some saying it was best for her and some saying she was just manipulative and not worth helping.

For me, everything changed when I started to work with Sharon in the community. I got to know her and how hard she was struggling with life. Her childhood had been rather grim; she was abused by her mother, bullied at school and raped whilst in her first job.

It was not easy for either of us; she always 'chose' to seriously self-harm at 5 p.m. on a Friday. Sharon and I persevered, though, and I started to believe she was trying and was willing to work on managing her emotions. I started to manage my emotions and frustrations and to give her the space she needed. That does not mean I did everything she demanded of me: we were very clear about what my boundaries were so I could maintain my well-being.

It was a long journey for Sharon (10 years after I first met her) and I only played a small, insignificant part for short periods; others with a similar attitude to mine took over when I moved on but I have had the privilege to see Sharon grow from the inpatient days to today. Sharon is now doing well. She has a full-time job, her own home and friends; she also has a crazy little car. I think Sharon has had a bigger impact on my life than I did on hers and I am very grateful.

Humanistic approaches, whether developmental, therapeutic or theoretical, offer care practitioners the opportunity to fully realise the person they are working with and the humanity within themselves. The case study of Daisy Dillon can be explored using all the developmental theories in this chapter. They could all offer an understanding of how she has come to be in the situation she is in and how she 'should' or 'could' be managed. This **management** will be explored in Chapter 7.

Biopsychologists

Biopsychologists may suggest that Sharon had a chemical imbalance, or hormonal or genetic problem.

Psychodynamic psychologists

Freud may suggest that, given her early life experiences, she has become fixated in one of the developmental stages and is using mental defence mechanisms to cope.

Erikson and Bowlby

Erikson may suggest that Sharon did not complete the first developmental crisis, which has led to a distrust in the world and problems for her achieving any of the other crises.

Bowlby would identify that Sharon did not develop a secure attachment with her mother, which has led to mental health problems in adult life and would predict that she will be unable to adequately care for her own children.

Behaviourists

Behaviourists would indicate that Sharon's problematic behaviour is due to early learning which has been reinforced into adulthood. She has learned the strategies of self-harm to manage her difficulties and she has not learned how to develop healthy relationships with others. This could be due to a lack of effective role models (social learning – Bandura), a lack of provision of rewards and punishment (operant conditioning – Skinner), or the association of pain receptors being stimulated with the release of endorphins (classical conditioning – Pavlov).

Cognitive psychologists

These would also implicate learning, but considering Piaget's theory, Sharon's environment has not offered her sufficient opportunities to reach her maturational milestones. She has not been able to achieve concrete operations.

Humanistic psychologists

These would indicate that Sharon has not been able to achieve her potential due to unfulfilled needs and the lack of positive regard. This has led to low self-esteem, anxiety, low moods and the inability to develop loving relationships as she is unable to love herself.

Chapter summary

This chapter has progressed from an exploration of the philosophical approaches that could be considered to underpin psychological developmental theories, particularly the empiricists (behaviourism, cognitivism, biologism) and the romanticists (psycho-dynamism, humanism). The staged developmental theories of Freud, Erikson, Bowlby and Piaget were examined and an overview of behaviourism, psychobiology and humanism was given. This was summed up with consideration of the case of Daisy Dillon.

Further study

The website of *Simply Psychology* offers detailed easy-to-read information on the nature/nurture debate and other issues in psychology. Its section on developmental psychology offers audiovisual recordings that will let you see the developmental theories in real life examples. See: www.simplypsychology.org/

Activity outline answers

Activity 2.1   Critical thinking

What do you think influences individual development? Do you think you are born to be the way you are or do you think that your environment shaped you – the nature/nurture debate?
   You may have identified:

- *Biological*: Genes, hormones, nutrition, exercise, sleep, physical contact
- *Sociological*: Family income, abuse, accommodation, education, health services
- *Psychological*: Attachment, comfort, stimulation, personal relationships
- *Spiritual*: Parents' belief system, religious rules, opportunity for play, access to open areas

Activity 2.3   Critical thinking

Bowlby said that only 60 per cent of mothers develop secure attachments with their children. What are the implications for society and care practitioners?
   If 40 per cent of children are at risk of becoming socially deviant or mentally ill, this can be a huge cost for society either by institutionalising people (prison/hospital) or by offering them social or healthcare. To reduce the need for treatment or detention of adults, society may decide to intervene when children are small – for example, by providing high-quality childcare and by giving parents the opportunity to stay with their children, for instance by maternity and paternity leave, staying in hospital with them, etc. Society could also decide to educate parents to enhance their parenting skills and monitor their performance. All of this can be seen to be done to differing levels within the UK. As care practitioners, we may be required to work with parents and babies, children and adults, who are struggling with their behaviour.

Activity 2.4   Critical thinking

Schema theory suggests that cognitive dissonance causes a person to reorganise their schema or stereotype of a person/incident/object, etc. How might you experience cognitive dissonance?

Cognitive dissonance is portrayed as psychological discomfort and may be experienced through stress reactions, such as lacking confidence in decisions or struggling with memory, attention or concentration. You might use mental defence mechanisms to reduce the dissonance, such as sublimating, rationalising or projecting, but the discomfort will need addressing eventually to return you to homeostasis.

References

Ainsworth, M. and Wittig, B.A. (1969) 'Attachment and exploratory behaviour of one-year-olds in a strange situation', in B.M. Foss (ed.), *Determinants of Infant Behaviour*, Vol. 4. London: Methuen, pp. 111–36.

Ainsworth, M.D.S., Blehar, M.C., Waters, E. and Wall, S. (1978) *Patterns of Attachment: A Psychological Study of the Strange Situation*. Hillsdale, NJ: Lawrence Erlbaum.

Barker, S. (2007) *Vital Notes for Nurses: Psychology*. Oxford: Blackwell.

Biro, F.M., Galvez, M.P. and Greenspan, L.C. (2010) 'Pubertal assessment method and baseline characteristics in a mixed longitudinal study of girls', *Paediatrics*. Published online, 9 August. Available at: www.ncbi.nlm.nih.gov/pubmed/20696727

Bowlby, J. (1951) 'Maternal care and mental health', *Bulletin of the World Health Organization*, 3: 355–534.

Davey, G. (2004) *Complete Psychology*. Oxford: Hodder and Stoughton.

Office for National Statistics (ONS) (2014) *Life Expectancy Tables*. Available at: http://ons.gov.uk/ons/rel/lifetables/national-life-tables/2010---2012/stb-uk-2010-2012.html (accessed June 2015).

Pierce, M. and Hardy, R. (2012) 'Commentary: The decreasing age of puberty – as much a psychosocial as a biological problem?', *International Journal of Epidemiology*, 41 (1): 300–2.

Stewart, W. (2013) *An A–Z of Counselling Theory and Practice*, 5th edn. Cheltenham: Nelson Thornes.

Willets, R.C., Gallop, A.P., Leandro, P.A., Lu, J.L.C., Macdonald, A.S., Miller, K.A., Richards, S.J., Robjohns, N., Ryan, J.P. and Waters, H.R. (2004) 'Longevity in the 21st century', *British Actuarial Journal*, 10: 685–832.

3 Understanding Suffering

Sue Barker

Suffering … Suffice

May all who suffer be sufficed

Let my strength support you

Let my touch comfort you

Let my words enfold you

May my presence bring you peace

May all who suffer be sufficed

Suffering … Suffice

Learning objectives

This chapter will develop an exploration of the psychological theories of health and illness, with a focus on suffering. The theories and research discussed in the chapter will provide a basis for the subsequent exploration of the psychological understanding of compassionate care as experienced by health and social care practitioners in order to enhance their performance. This chapter's learning objectives are to:

- Describe the psychological theories of health and illness
- Discuss the meaning of suffering and how it is experienced
- Recognise how Carper's aesthetic, personal, ethical and empirical ways of knowing can, alongside intuitive knowledge, help your understanding of suffering

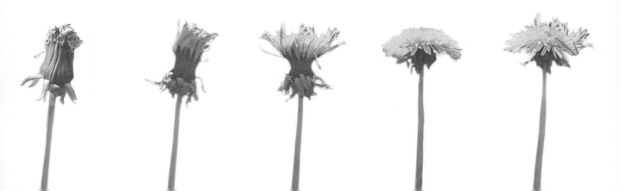

Activity 3.1   Reflection

Spend a few minutes thinking about what health means to you:

- Is it something to do with not being physically or mentally ill?
- Is it something to do with how you feel?
- Is it to do with what you can do?

As this is a reflection, there is no outline answer at the end of the chapter.

Health

The English word 'health' comes from the Old English (Anglo-Saxon) word *hale*, meaning 'wholeness, being whole, sound or well'. *Hale* comes from the Proto-Indo-European root *kailo*, meaning 'whole, uninjured, of good omen'. 'Holy' has the same root, and we have in the past seen a close link between 'health' and 'holy', with mediaeval monks providing both spiritual and physical care to enhance health. We can also find this link in some contemporary cultures where the shaman provides both spiritual and medical guidance. If we reconsider the definition of psychology in Chapter 1, we find a similar link with spirituality, *psyche* meaning 'mind' or 'spirit'. It is therefore interesting that psychological theories and health theories rarely include this element of health or psyche.

As with many terms, 'health' can be interpreted in different ways by different groups of people at different times: there is some cultural element to its definition. This makes a precise definition problematic. Health psychologists usually adopt what has been called a **biopsychosocial** model of health. It is an approach that views disease and symptoms as being determined by physical, social and psychological factors. This model can be seen in most contemporary definitions of health.

Probably the most famous definition of health is: '*Health is a state of complete physical, mental and social well-being and not merely the absence of disease or infirmity,*' delivered by the World Health Organization (WHO, 1948: 100). This definition has not been amended since 1948, but there have been many additional explanations of health by the WHO and other interested organisations. *The Lancet*, a prestigious medical journal, published an article questioning the WHO definition which asserts that health is not a 'state of complete physical, mental, and social well-being'. They stress that with new understandings at a molecular, individual and societal level of illness and disease, the definition needs to be changed.

Despite the continuing acceptance of the above WHO definition during the Ottawa Charter for Health Promotion in 1986, the WHO developed their explanation of health by stating that it is: '*a resource for everyday life, not the objective of living. Health is a positive concept emphasizing social and personal resources, as well as physical capacities*' (WHO, 1986).

In 2011, the UK Government developed a number of cross-governmental strategies focused on health, such as the 'Global Health Outcomes Framework' and 'No Health without Mental Health'. The Global Health Strategy was updated in 2014 (Public Health England, 2014). This new strategy identifies the problems with defining health and what this might mean in a global arena, so they accepted the definition developed by the group in 2008:

> Global health: refers to health issues where the determinants circumvent, undermine or are oblivious to the territorial boundaries of states, and are thus beyond the capacity of individual countries to address through domestic institutions. Global health is focused on people across the whole planet rather than the concerns of particular nations. Global health recognises that health is determined by problems, issues and concerns that transcend national boundaries. (Public Health England, 2014: 7).

This definition again does not recognise the relevance of spirituality, but both the WHO and the UK Government provide accounts that accept a biopsychosocial model of health as outlined by health psychologists. Health psychologists are people who have studied psychology and then developed their career to focus on health. They apply 'psychological methods to the study of behaviour relevant to health, illness and healthcare' (NHS Careers, 2015). They also integrate different theoretical perspectives (cognitive, developmental and social) to understand the phenomenon of health and how to improve it. Given that the primary focus of psychology is developing a scientific understanding of people, this is the philosophical approach, the empirical approach, undertaken by health psychologists. They explore individual health behaviour and what guides that, along with community or interactional influences on health (Morrison and Bennett, 2012).

The biopsychosocial model adopted by health psychologists leads them to seek to understand what impacts on health for the individual, social groups and societies. In 1961, Bauman, the health psychologist, attempted to find out what the general public thought health was by asking people. She found that the responses fell into three categories. Health is:

- A general sense of well-being
- The absence of symptoms of disease
- Things that a physically fit person can do

These relate to feeling, symptom orientation and performance.

Activity 3.2   Reflection

Return to your understanding of what health means to you. Does your definition fall into one, two or all three of these categories or does it highlight something very different?

As this is a reflection, there is no outline answer at the end of the chapter.

It is acknowledged, though, that how an individual describes health is reactive to their current health status. A large study (Blaxter, 1990) went on to ascertain social views of health and they found that:

- Health as not ill
- Health as reserve
- Health as behaviour
- Health as physical fitness or vitality
- Health as psychosocial well-being
- Health as function

Understandings of health are also determined by age or lifespan and change not only with time but also with learning, experience and maturation. Health psychologists facilitate our understanding that the term 'health' refers to some sort of objective assessment whereas 'well-being' refers to a subjective assessment or the individual's feelings.

Well-being

Contemporary society has moved towards a focus on well-being rather than health per se, with both social and healthcare defining it and encouraging practice to work towards it. The Social Care Institute of Excellence (SCIE) (2005) identify that well-being refers to our subjective assessment of how we feel about our life experiences. The Department of Health (2007: 99) offers the following definition:

> Well-being is the subjective state of being healthy, happy, contented, comfortable and satisfied with one's quality of life. It includes physical, material, social, emotional ('happiness'), and development and activity dimensions.

Well-being does not appear to **correlate** with physical health as the oldest and youngest within society have the highest rates of well-being but older people also have the highest rates of physical ill health (Barker, 2013).

Within psychology, the humanistic perspective has led to a greater exploration of well-being through the work of Rogers and Maslow (Barker, 2007). Further progress in the humanistic movement, along with anthropology and developments in phenomenological thinking, facilitated the development of Tom Kitwood's (1997) person-centred care for people with dementia and Todres et al.'s (2009) humanisation of care.

Kitwood and Bredin (1992: 281–2) recognises a state of well-being as when a person is able to:

- Assert their desire or will
- Express a range of emotions
- Initiate social contact
- Experience affectional warmth
- Experience social sensitivity
- Experience **self-respect**
- Experience acceptance
- Express humour

- Be creative and express themselves
- Show pleasure
- Be helpful
- Experience relaxation

Within care, this is achieved through a culture of **positive person work** and absence of **malignant social psychology**. There are a number of approaches that facilitate a conducive environment for well-being; these include a humanised approach (Todres et al., 2009) and person-centred care or positive person work (Kitwood, 1997). Kitwood suggests that dominant cultures are difficult to change, but that the culture of dementia care needs to change in order to provide person-centred care to achieve well-being (Kitwood, 1997). Todres et al. (2009) also recognise the need for cultural change to facilitate well-being within caring services.

Kitwood (1997) identifies the psychological requirements for the person to achieve well-being. These are: attachment, occupation, identity, inclusion, comfort and the overarching need for love. Kitwood offers the figure of a flower to help visualise these needs (see Figure 3.1).

These needs clearly link with the needs established by Maslow but also fit well with the romantic and psychodynamic theories of development. The romantic and psychodynamic theorists also state that for a person to become whole, to have personal integrity and a secure self-concept, they need to develop attachment, belonging, skill (occupation) and love. Kitwood particularly states the need for **personhood**, which he articulates as something that is bestowed on a person by their culture through relationships with others. If the person does not gain a sense of personhood, they become depersonalised or in Todres et al.'s (2009) terminology, 'dehumanised'.

Therefore – for the humanists Rogers and Maslow and psychodynamicists Freud, Erikson and Bowlby – the person needs a holistic sense of well-being which has **intrapersonal, interpersonal and extrapersonal** elements. This also appears to be the case for the more recent theories associated with well-being, such as Kitwood's person-centred care and Todres et al.'s humanising of care (these will be explored in more detail in Chapter 5).

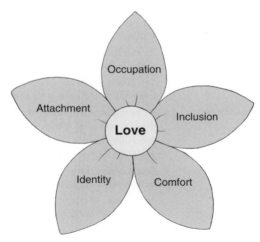

Figure 3.1 Flower of needs

Illness or ill-being

Ill-being for Kitwood is the opposite of well-being and occurs in a culture of malignant social psychology encouraging dependence and self-deprecation which can lead to low self-esteem, anxiety and depression. Ill-being is therefore a lack of personhood, preventing people from achieving well-being. In the care situation, ill-being occurs in a culture of malignant social psychology.

Activity 3.3   Reflection

Spend a few moments to consider what ill-being might mean for you.

As this is a reflection, there is no outline answer at the end of the chapter.

What malignant social psychology involves is shown in Table 3.1.

Table 3.1   Kitwood's 17 malignancies (1997)

Malignancy	Definition and example
Treachery	This is where you manipulated the person to comply with your wishes; e.g. the person states that they would like a drink and you say: 'If you come with me, I will get you a drink,' but you actually take them to the bathroom
Disempowerment	This is where you reduce the person's ability to take control. An example could be where the person is able to use a fork but you only provide them with a spoon
Infantilisation	This is treating an adult as if they were a small child. An example could be that when giving a person their lunch, you say: 'There we go, you eat that all up like a good girl and don't spill it down yourself'
Intimidation	This situation could be seen to occur if you say to a person who was walking to the door: 'Don't you dare go out of that door or I will take your shoes and coat away'
Labelling	An example could be that a person is noisily seeking attention and you explain to a visitor: 'Oh, that is just because of the dementia'
Stigmatisation	An example could be that when talking to another person about working in a particular area, you state: 'Oh you don't want to work there: they are all demented down there'
Outpacing	This is where you are working at a pace that is too fast for the person, e.g. giving information too quickly for them to understand
Invalidation	An example of this could be where the person says that they are unhappy and you say: 'No you are not: it is a lovely sunny day, which makes you happy'
Banishment	This could occur if you are sitting reading notes and the person comes up to you, and you take them to the day room and walk off, shutting the door behind you
Objectification	This is where the person is treated as if they were an object, e.g. they are sat in a wheelchair and suddenly moved to another area without explanation
Ignoring	An example of this is where two carers are sat talking to each other across the person without acknowledging that they are there
Imposition	This is forcing the person to do something that they do not want to do, such as turning the television on in the room when they did not want to watch it
Withholding	This can be seen when a person is requesting a drink but this is being ignored
Accusation	This is blaming the person when they were unable to change the situation; e.g. a drink is put by their side for another person and they drink it, as they believe that it is for them
Disruption	This can be seen to occur when the person is in the middle of reminiscing about something from their past and you interrupt and change the subject
Mockery	This is where the carer laughs or makes derogatory comments at the behaviour exhibited by the person
Disparagement	This occurs when you make a negative comment to the person, such as: 'You are being really difficult today,' which can lower self-esteem

Ill-being can be seen as a psychological or emotional experience and leads to emotional suffering and, as with well-being, can be considered to be more subjective than health or illness.

Illness has been referred to as the individual experiencing a feeling of not being normal or right, of something being wrong, and disease has been understood as the label which doctors have given to this 'not rightness'. Definitions of illness are accepted as more objective than the rather subjective definition of ill-being. Illness is seen as a period of disease or sickness which affects the body or mind. Health psychologists have identified that health and illness identification are influenced by the person's prior experience of illness, their understanding of medical knowledge, and whether they are an expert or a lay person. A 'common-sense' model of illness which provides illness prototypes is based on identity (the experienced symptoms), the perceived cause, consequences, timeline (how long it might last), the cure and the type of person experiencing the 'illness'. These personal prototypes then lead to health-related behaviours. People can also use others' illness prototypes to guide their health-seeking behaviour (Morrison and Bennett, 2012).

 ## David Smith

David is 64 years old and a farmer. He started helping his father on the farm as a child and has felt farming to be his vocation. David is rarely ill and has had no major health problems. He was physically fit and strong and had an optimistic worldview, despite having to deal with tragedies such as his whole herd of cows being slaughtered due to tuberculosis infection.

David started to become excessively fatigued, had a headache and was shivery. He believed this was caused by a virus and that if he took some painkillers he could get on with his work. If David did not get on with his animal care, the animals would lose their condition, which would have long-term consequences for David and the animals. David thought he would only need to take painkillers for a day or two and that his body would then restore itself to health.

 ## Isobel Jones

Isobel is 30 years old and a primary school teacher. She has always enjoyed working with children and grew up in a home where there were extra children around as her parents were foster parents as well as her and her sibling's birth parents. When she was a child, if she or any of the other children were unwell her mother would tuck them up in bed or sit them on the settee under a blanket. Her mother would bring her warm drinks and would gently stroke her hair.

Isobel started to become excessively fatigued, had a headache and was shivery. She believed that this was caused by a virus and so she needed to tuck herself up in bed with a warm drink: she also repeatedly tucked her hair behind her ears in a self-stroking motion. Isobel thought that if she went into work with a virus, she would pass it on to the children, and given that she was extremely fatigued she would not be able to be as patient as she should be with them. Isobel thought she would only need to rest for a day or two and that her body would then restore itself to health.

Case study

Case study

In the case studies of David and Isobel, their individual illness prototypes have many similarities but their behaviours are different. We can see that early life experiences have led to Isobel self-caring and showing herself compassion but David demonstrated the need to be stoic. Neither of them chose to seek medical advice as they believed that their ill health would be rectified by their own bodies. If, as David and Isobel thought, they had a minor virus that would be dealt with by their bodies in a couple of days, neither of their health behaviours would be a problem. If the symptoms experienced by them were indicators of a more serious condition, Isobel's health behaviour should not increase its progression but David's behaviour might.

Health psychologists use a psychosocial model for understanding health and health behaviours. This facilitates their providing social and healthcare practitioners with information to care for people experiencing health problems and to enhance their well-being.

Alongside the genesis of health psychology as an academic discipline, other associated interdisciplinary approaches have been developing. One that is mentioned in a number of health psychology texts is psychoneuroimmunology.

Psychoneuroimmunology

The interaction between different organs and systems in the body has been explored for hundreds of years, but in 1975 Ader (a psychologist) and Cohen (an immunologist) coined the term 'psychoneuroimmunology' based on their experimental work with animals. Psychoneuroimmunology is the study of the interaction between psychology ('psycho'), neurology ('neuro') and immunology.

The nervous system sends chemical messengers in the form of neurotransmitters. Some of these are released into organs which form part of the immune system, and the immune system then releases hormones which influence the nervous system. A good example where this can be seen to work is in the experience of stress.

When a person experiences stress it is usually initially perceived by the senses, but people can perceive stress from memories or their imagination. Perception is recognised as a psychological process. This psychological perception of stress activates the **hypothalamus** in the brain, which has **neuroendocrine cells** which release corticotropin-releasing hormone (CRH). This activates the **pituitary gland**, which is part of the brain but also part of the immune system.

The pituitary gland secretes adrenocorticotropic **hormone** which activates the adrenal glands (immune system) that sit above the kidneys. The adrenal glands secrete **corticosteroids**, which increase metabolism of sugars, proteins and fats. If this continues for an excessive amount of time it can lead to metabolic disorders such as diabetes. Corticosteroids inhibit the macrophages, helper T cells and effector cells in the immune system too. The adrenal glands also release a **neurotransmitter** called **adrenaline**.

Adrenaline prepares the body to deal with stressors, causing blood to be diverted to the major muscle groups, and increases blood pressure. If this continues for an excessive amount of time, the person may experience cardiovascular problems such as high blood pressure and atherosclerosis. There will also be behavioural changes in responses to internal and external events (psychological responses).

This interactional pathway is known as the **hypothalamic–pituitary–adrenal axis (HPA axis)** (see Figure 3.2).

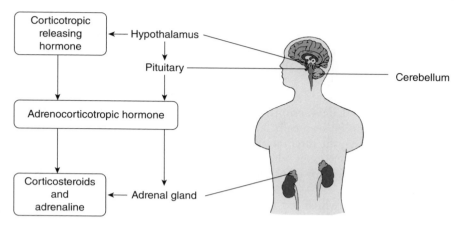

Figure 3.2 The hypothalamic–pituitary–adrenal axis (HPA axis)

This is just a brief overview of one system demonstrating the link between psychology, neurology and immunology. This can help care practitioners develop an understanding of the need to recognise people who they are working with in a holistic person-centred way.

The next section is going to explore suffering, which is seen as the outcome of ill-being or illness. Given the symbiotic relationship between all parts of the human body, including the mind, it is important that all of these are considered when exploring the impact and amelioration of illness and ill-being.

Suffering

Activity 3.4 Reflection

What does suffering mean to you? What would you be experiencing to identify it as suffering?

As this is a reflection, there is no outline answer at the end of the chapter.

Suffering has been explored by philosophers and theologians over the centuries, and as with all terms related to human experience, it is influenced by the prevailing culture. It has been explored through religious (Buddhism, Hinduism, Christianity, Islam), philosophical (Epicurus, Nietzsche, Frankl), moral (Bentham, 1988) and ethical (Parse, 2010) lenses as well as the social sciences, including psychology (particularly Freud and Rogers). Bentham (1988) highlights that it is a state of being which all sentient creatures may experience.

Psychologists have been interested in suffering as a human phenomenon since the late nineteenth century. Their exploration and understanding of it have been shaped by the philosophical underpinning of their view of people, which also allows for their categorisation into certain psychological perspectives. Some psychologists recognise suffering as an internal phenomenon – as would be expected of the romantics such as Freud or Rogers. Others view it as an evolutionary, Darwinian, adaptive trait or learned behaviour, both of which focus on its ability to protect the person and offer coping strategies for trauma, injury or distress.

Biopsychologists, through brain-scanning, offer explanations of the link between suffering and psychosocial interactions. Given that it has been found that the cingulate cortex in the brain can be seen to be electronically active during times of both physical and emotional suffering, the interaction between physical and psychological functioning is closely related. This was seen when exploring psychoneuroimmunology (PNI) but it also offers a rationalisation for using psychosocial interventions or interactions to reduce suffering.

The Enlightenment – which led to many changes in how people understood themselves and their world – as would be expected, influenced the understanding of suffering. Post-Enlightenment in the eighteenth and nineteenth centuries, a generally positive model of suffering was accepted, in line with Frankl's (1963) statement that suffering involves finding meaning in life. In the nineteenth and twentieth centuries, society saw an increase in medicalisation, bureaucratisation and secularism. As with health, we can see a gradual movement in this time, from a spiritual understanding of suffering to a medical viewpoint.

Davies (2011) outlines three positive models of suffering in the nineteenth and twentieth centuries: the Christian, romantic and Freudian. The Christian model acknowledged an interplay between spirit and suffering. The spirit is the person's link with God: they experience God through an intimacy with the Holy Spirit of God. Suffering plays an intrinsic part in this relationship. The person needs to acknowledge their sinfulness and suffer the feeling of inadequacy so that God can save them through the suffering of his Son. People go through suffering to become better people and achieve holiness. Christians see suffering as a path to moral and spiritual development, which is clearly seen in their rallying cry of Jesus saying to his disciples: 'Pick up your cross and follow me.'

The romantic movement was discussed in Chapter 2 and is the second model. The third positive model that Davies (2011) offers is a Freudian one. We identified that Freud had much in common with the romantics but Davies, acknowledging the differences, puts the romantic philosophical approach and the Freudian psychological approach into separate models.

The romantics recognised a superficial level of the person as well as a deep level from which creative abilities grew and bubbled to the surface, superficial level. They were concerned that contemporary society's bureaucracy, industrialisation and secularisation were interfering with the person's ability to express their creativity and engage with their deeper level. Without this engagement, the person could not fully experience nature, nor deep joy or sorrow. Suffering was seen as positive and necessary as it makes people sensitive to the destructive elements of nature, leading to wisdom, and facilitates **empathy** with others which leads to compassion.

Freud is probably the most influential theorist linking suffering and human change. Davies offers Freud's psychological theory as his third model. Freud identified that, through suffering, people move from a state of being unconscious of their motivations to having a conscious awareness. He identified these unconscious motivations as being a threat to the person's integrity. Freud suggested that when suffering became observable, the person was on the path to recovery. This was because mental defence mechanisms which hid the person's real motivations were being dismantled, allowing the person to develop conscious understanding. Freud offered the analogy that this process was like surgery without anaesthetic.

Whilst Davies (2011) recognises the positive nature of Freud's view of suffering, Eriksson (2014) identifies how **psychoanalysis** (explored in more detail in Chapter 7), the therapy provided by Freud's theory, provides the path through suffering to freedom. Rather than seeing this as a psychological or medical cure, he indicates that it offers a moral cure. The bringing-to-consciousness of harmful, immoral motivations allows the person to liberate themselves from these motivations and mental defence mechanisms that hold them in the unconscious mind.

Another psychologist who explored suffering was Carl Rogers, although it is not presented as such. Rogers' theory grew out of a turning-away from Freud's psychodynamic approach and behaviourism whilst accepting some elements of these. Rogers accepted both an internal motivation (**unique potential**) as well as external or environmental influences identified by the behaviourists (the need for unconditional positive regard). His **client-centred therapy**, now known as **person-centred care**, which will be referred to throughout this book, was developed to offer people the personal space to recognise their individual potential and facilitate their becoming themselves through therapeutic relationships. For Rogers, suffering is a negative experience. He identified people growing through self-recognition and unconditional positive regard. People suffer if they are trying to be what others expect of them, using what he called the **organismic valuing process** (**OVP**). They are not growing towards their potential – towards what Maslow called self-actualisation.

Over the last 30 years, understanding of suffering has radically changed from a mostly positive model (suffering has a purpose) to a negative one (suffering is purposeless). This shift can be seen in psychological views of suffering, too: Freud's theory offered a positive model of suffering, whereas Rogers' can be seen as negative. Davies (2011: 188) states that this was due to the 'rationalisation of suffering' through its repositioning in medicine (biology and psychiatry) rather than spirituality, philosophy or morals. This leads to the expectation that healthcare workers will reduce or ameliorate it (Milton, 2013).

Within contemporary culture, suffering is seen as the undergoing of pain or distress, and linked to this is the etymological root of 'patient': to suffer. 'To suffer' comes from the Latin word *sufferre* (*ferre* – meaning 'to bear' or 'endure'). Current theorists such as Johnston (2013: 230) offer definitions that incorporate some philosophical understanding but couched within a contemporary negative model: 'suffering involves the loss of acceptable meaning and nourishing connection'. However, there are still some people in society today who recognise suffering as having a positive role, for example Harris (2007), with the assertion that the 'gift' of suffering can increase compassion in others. Rehnsfeldt and Eriksson (2004) offer a way of bringing together these two poles. They state that it is whether suffering is bearable or unbearable that indicates its positivity or negativity. If suffering is bearable it can lead to personal understanding and development but, if it is unbearable, understanding of self and life is removed, leaving a darkness.

Suffering is frequently a topic of conversation in healthcare literature, particularly as reduction of suffering is now seen as part of the role of care professionals. Rehnsfeldt and Eriksson (2004) lead carers to engage in true compassion, to share the experience of the other person, to make unbearable suffering bearable. Through this caring relation-ship, carer and sufferer can both gain a better understanding of themselves and the meaning of their life: **ontology**.

Activity 3.5 Reflection

Think back to the previous reflection when you considered what suffering was for you. Did it include positive elements or were they all negative? Do you think it is the role of nurses to reduce suffering?

As this is a reflection, there is no outline answer at the end of the chapter.

Janice Morse, a nurse, and her colleagues have been studying suffering for over 15 years. Their approach is one that focuses on behaviour so it could be considered empirical but she uses a *qualitative research paradigm*. Morse et al. (1994) suggest that suffering causes the person to focus on the **corporeal** and inhibits their ability to engage with personal meaning or interaction with others. This appears to be what Eriksson has identified as unbearable suffering. She goes on to describe two types of suffering: emotional releasing and enduring suffering (Morse, 2000).

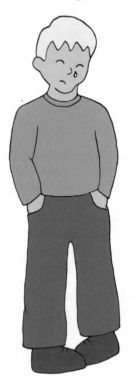

Enduring suffering is where a person shuts off their emo-tions to cope, whereas emotional suffering is where a person releases their emotions. Enduring suffering is where a person is protecting themselves from suffering whereas emotional releasing is where the person is emotionally responding to the experience. Contemporary carers tend to believe that it is nor-mal to respond to suffering by expressing emotions, but in the past we can find examples of where children and men are encouraged to hold their emotions and not to 'cry' or 'cry out' (Figure 3.3).

Morse and her colleagues (1994, 1995, 2000, 2001) focused on developing a theory of suffering gained from the experiences of patients and nurses. They appear to have linked the terms 'suffering' and 'discomfort', both identified as having a corpo-real focus (Morse et al., 1994), but others suggest that discom-fort differs and state that it has mind, body and spiritual elements (Schuiling and Sampselle, 1999).

A person's awareness of their body when well or comfortable is limited, but when they are in discomfort or suffering this changes and they become acutely conscious of their body and themselves. Nine themes of discomfort have been found: dis-eased body, disobedient body, deceiving body, vulnerable body, violated body, enduring body, betraying body, resigned body and betraying mind. This was established by interviewing patients who had experienced extreme pain or discomfort and

Figure 3.3 Being brave traumatic injuries or life-threatening illness (Morse et al., 1994).

Laura, Carol and Peter – Part 1

Laura has recently moved back into the family home, with her mother, Carol, and father, Peter, after her relationship with her partner broke down. Her brother is still at university. Fortunately Laura could continue to work in her current post but it meant an extended commute. Laura was struggling with her feelings and very easily became tearful especially after working all day and a long commute home. Laura's mother worked full time but worked near to the house and so she undertook the entire housework and cooking for the family. Laura's father is on sick leave from work as he was recently diagnosed with multiple sclerosis and is experiencing pain in his feet, blurred vision and tingling in his hands and arms. He makes a joke of being at home, encouraging Laura to believe that he does not need to be at home and that he is fit enough to be at work, but work managers are being difficult about his return.

In the case study of Laura, we can see that all three members of the family are suffering. They could all be considered to be trying to use enduring suffering as a way of managing but sometimes Laura cannot achieve this and reverts to emotional release. Peter may be experiencing several areas of suffering: diseased body, disobedient body, deceiving body and vulnerable body. Carol could also be experiencing suffering in terms of enduring body and resigned body whereas Laura's experiences may be labelled betraying body and betraying mind.

Morse and her colleagues, after developing this understanding of suffering, went on to identify effective caring responses to reduce suffering or to make it bearable. Linking suffering with discomfort, they recognised these caring responses as providing comfort. Morse et al. (1994) highlight through their research that for care practitioners to achieve total comfort is unattainable but to enhance comfort to ease and relieve distress is a central element of their role.

Comfort

A state of comfort in the mind involves a feeling of peace and security, and freedom from anxiety or worry. Within the body it involves physical needs being met, such as hunger, thirst, sleep, air and freedom from illness, whereas spiritual comfort involves a feeling of hope and expectation, transcendence from pain and being at one with one's god (Barker, 2011). The assessment of comfort needs and the provision of comfort by carers should include all aspects of the person as they are interrelated (see Chapters 4 and 5).

Morse and her colleagues state that different approaches are required to provide comfort for those suffering, depending on what type of suffering they are experiencing. When a person is demonstrating enduring suffering, to provide comfort at this time carers use strategies to support endurance by showing respect for the person. Strategies usually accessed at this stage are encouragement and praise, whereas when a person is suffering and emotionally responding to their situation, caregivers physically support the person by hugging, holding and extensively using touch.

Morse et al. (1994) stress that it is not the activity of care that is important: it is the way in which it is undertaken. If it is undertaken 'for' and 'with' the person, instead of 'to' the person, it restores their integrity and assists in moving them towards recovery.

This would also appear to be the aim of person-centred care. When the anticipation of pain, whether physical or emotional, cannot be removed the caregiver can offer comfort by protecting, bolstering and advocating for the person (Morse et al., 1994).

Case study

 ## Laura, Carol and Peter – Part 2

Carol had arrived home from work and had started to cook the evening meal for them all. She was tired and her feet ached but she felt she must care for her family. Peter was lying on the bed upstairs: he had not slept well the previous night and was trying to manage the pain in his feet. Carol understood his pain and his concern about the future and had tried to offer him comfort by listening to him, acknowledging his discomfort and offering to get pain relief and a hot drink for him. Peter became cross at her suggested actions as he had already tried these without relief. Carol had spent some time telling him how much she loved him and how he was coping much better than she would in his situation. She sat with him and gave him the space to talk, just giving small encouragements to continue until he had said all he had energy for. She then left him to rest with a gentle kiss on his cheek.

Carol had almost finished cooking when Laura arrived home. Laura had had a difficult day as her ex-partner had been in the coffee shop that she had gone to for lunch with a colleague and he had come over and spoken to her colleague and ignored her. She then had a difficult customer who shouted at her, and the journey home had taken longer than usual due to heavy traffic. Laura came in to the kitchen and cried. Carol stopped cooking and put her arms around her daughter and hugged her tight. She did not use any words: she just held her until her daughter had finished sobbing.

Despite Carol's personal suffering and her need to give comfort she provided a meal for her family and when they were able to sit together later to watch television she sat in between Laura and Peter and felt comfortable.

In the case study, Carol can be seen to be providing care for and with Peter and Laura. She provided the environment for Peter to express his emotions and then to regain control of himself and return to an enduring suffering which he felt more comfortable with. Carol can be seen to help both Peter and Laura from a state of unbearable suffering to bearable suffering. Once Peter and Laura returned to bearable suffering, Carol showed them respect and allowed them to give and share comfort with her; they were compassionate with each other.

The provision of comfort is undertaken in a number of ways but extensively involves the carer using their whole self. This use of self includes being present or connected to the other person. Carers achieve this connection through the use of their hands, eyes and voices using '**comfort talk register**, eye contact and touch' (Morse, 2001: 52). Through their hands, eyes and voices they can facilitate rapport, understanding, control and hope (Figure 3.4).

Most texts that explore the necessary skills to achieve comfort and provide care identify the need for the carer to be **empathetic**. Empathy is where the carer understands the other person's experiences and can demonstrate this understanding to them. According to the humanists such as Rogers, there are four core conditions to therapy or therapeutic communication: empathy, genuineness or congruence, warmth and unconditional positive regard. A general adoption of psychological approaches by carers in general can, however, be problematic (Morse et al., 1992). An unquestioning adoption of, and pressure to engage with, the concept of empathy may create too great a burden on carers. This might then lead to ill-health or avoidance of care by the professional (Morse et al., 1992). If we return to the case study of Laura, Carol and Peter we can easily see that Carol may find herself becoming over-burdened, leading to either avoidance of Laura and Peter, or she may develop health problems herself.

Empathetic insight can lead to the carer embodying the suffering of the other so that they are not only responsible for alleviating the

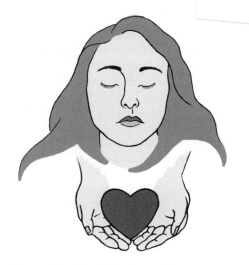

Figure 3.4   Head, hands and heart

suffering of the person but also experiencing it as they provide care. To a certain extent, this is inevitable as carers work in close and intimate ways with those they care for. It may be that intentionally seeking this type of experience does not offer comfort to the sufferer and may damage the carer. This emotional involvement may reduce their ability to care and create an additional **emotional labour** (further explored in Chapter 9) for them and lead to **burnout**. Morse et al. (1992), in contrast to other caring texts, go on to suggest that there may be a role for **sympathy** in caring.

Sympathy is the expression of the carer's emotions in response to the sufferer. Whilst this is a problem if it puts an emotional burden on the sufferer it can legitimise the suffering being experienced and allow the person to care for themselves. It can also demonstrate acceptance of the person's suffering if demonstrated in a genuine manner at an appropriate time (Morse et al., 1992).

This raises the question of how the care practitioner knows what approach to suffering they need to use and when. Morse offers some guidance based on enduring suffering, emotional releasing and the nine types of suffering but it is difficult to assess which type of suffering a person may be experiencing in the practice situation.

Ways of knowing

Barbara Carper (1978) established four ways or patterns of knowing in nursing, which she called empirical, personal, ethical and aesthetic.

- *Empirical*: As already explored, this is the understanding of knowledge derived from the scientific approach
- *Personal*: This is the knowledge, understanding and attitudes developed from self-knowledge or understanding. It is most closely linked to self-understanding through empathy of another person's experience. It is knowledge that can be gained through imagining you are in another person's position to understand their particular experience

- *Ethical*: Ethics are closely linked to morals but ethical frameworks are usually developed in the professional arena whereas morals are seen as more personal. This way of knowing is about exploring and understanding the experience or situation through questioning of choices and their consequences. The ability to judge the best choice based on an exploration of the decision uses an ethical framework
- *Aesthetic*: This term is usually used to refer to consideration of art and beauty but here it is about the sensing or perceiving of something and might be labelled intuition

To explore and understand suffering and how to respond to it, all of these ways of knowing could be helpful. Empirically, there have been a number of questionnaires and psychometric tests used to assess suffering. These include the Edmonton Symptom Assessment System, measures of spiritual well-being and despair and of pain assessment that take into account nonverbal indicators of suffering (Schulz et al., 2007). Personal knowing of suffering could be gained through the care practitioners' personal experiences. All people experience suffering at some point in their lives. A knowledge and memory of this can guide the care practitioner's interactions to develop empathy for the other person. Through **self-awareness** and empathy, personal knowing will grow and support their practice (see Chapters 6 and 7).

An ethical or moral way of knowing about suffering could be gained through reflective practices, which are seen as an essential element of professional practice in care. Reflective models guide practitioners to question their understanding and application of knowledge to their practice. Within this reflective practice, ethical frameworks can be applied, for example the biomedical ethical principles of beneficence, non-maleficence, autonomy and justice. There are other ethical frameworks, such as provided by the Nuffield ethical principles in dementia care and professional codes of practice, British Psychological Society, Nursing Midwifery Council, Health and Care Professions Council (HCPC) and the General Social Care Council.

Aesthetic ways of knowing tend to be less highly regarded in professional practice, with some professions indicating that practitioners should only use evidence-based practice (EBP) which is hierarchically categorised by government. Evidence-based practice provides the empirical way of knowing but Carper suggests that there is a need for aesthetic ways of knowing, too. Whilst it is easy to see that to base care practices on how something 'looks', if it is artistic or beautiful, is of limited use, deeper consideration of aesthetics is useful to care practitioners. As individuals we frequently assess things by asking 'Do they feel right?' or 'Does this look comfortable?' or 'Does it look okay?'

 Lucy Thomas

Case study

Lucy was a 93-year-old lady I had been caring for in a nursing home. The home is excellent and has received awards for its care practices and for its staff development. Lucy had been at the home for some time. She was a quiet lady who enjoyed watching the passers-by through the window and despite not enjoying joining in with the group activities she was happy to sit and watch. Lucy needed some support with personal care but this was not an issue for her. She had a close family who regularly visited her and I would consider her to have a high quality of life. The nurse had been in to give her her medicine and to do her medical checks and had told me everything was fine. I went into Lucy's room to see if she wanted to join the others in the day room as it was the coffee morning that Lucy usually enjoyed, as she would sit and knit and listen to everyone's stories. This morning, Lucy was polite and smiled as usual but I knew something was not right. I asked her if she was alright and she said yes but things just did not feel right. I do not know why, but instead of walking Lucy to the day room I sat and looked out of the window with her and she held my hand. As we sat there peaceably, after only a few minutes her breathing became quieter and she closed her eyes. She was not to open them again.

If we consider the case study of Lucy Thomas, we can see an example of aesthetic knowing, of which there are many within all areas of health and social care. The care practitioner gains some understanding that they are unable to pinpoint the origin of, but this guides their practice.

Carper's ways of knowing provide a framework to explore a situation or experience in greater depth and to move away from a purely scientific or empirical way of knowing. She facilitated with this work the development of reflective practice and an acknowledgment that caring is an art, not just a science, in the same way that Freud and Rogers have done with psychological understanding. She also opened more widely the exploration of the use of the aesthetic or intuition in care.

Patricia Benner (1984) in her seminal book *From Novice to Expert* clearly identified that expert nurses use their intuition in the caring practices. She further develops her explanation to identify that, as practitioners develop experience, their conscious knowledge of practice becomes tacit. They move from unconscious incompetence (novice) to unconscious competence (expert). She went on to label this 'patterning' (Benner et al., 2010).

Carper's aesthetic way of knowing has been further developed by a number of writers using a number of terms: 'intuition' (Morse et al., 1994; Davis-Floyd and Davis, 1996), 'tacit knowing and knowledge' (Benner and Wrubel, 1989), 'embodied knowledge' (Polkinghorne, 2004), 'reflexivity and reflection in action' (Johns, 1995, 2000, 2013) and 'emotional intelligence' (Goleman, 1998).

Benner and Wrubel (1989) described intuition as how we 'know how', which they identify as tacit knowledge or knowledge that lacks an explanation but is relational; it is embedded in the situation. Hildingsson and Häggström (1999) referred to intuition as an interpretive tool used by midwives as a means to identify the needs of women, in a similar way to the nurses in Morse et al.'s study (1994). Johns (2000) advocated reflection as a process for uncovering this tacit knowing or knowledge which he recognised as intuition.

Three ways of intuitive-knowing have been identified:

- *Intuition based on practice experience*: This can be seen to refer to where practitioners develop an inner knowing through experience and may be what Benner is suggesting in her expert nurses
- *Intuition based on spiritual awareness*: This appears to be where the practitioner received a word or message, which could be a vision that is accounted for as a spiritual experience
- *Intuition based on connectiveness*: Practitioners are using their intimate knowledge of the person to understand them, their needs and their possible outcomes.

These different types of intuition, though, are seen to be overlapping and interrelated (Ólafsdóttir, 2009).

Intuition based on connectiveness is 'an awareness creating relationship' or 'tuning in' (Ólafsdóttir, 2009) providing a 'relational way of understanding or knowing' (Todres, 2008). This is a way of knowing that is related to the life world and is concerned with relationships and connection. It establishes a concrete relationship between carer and cared for as part of a living situation (Todres, 2008).

Chapter summary

This chapter has explored what health, illness, ill-being and well-being might be, gaining the understanding that health tends to refer to an objective assessment and well-being a more subjective assessment of the person's status. This was followed by a discussion of what suffering might be and how it might be experienced. Suffering could be seen to be both outward signs of discomfort and emotional releasing as well as an enduring of suffering, a holding of the feeling inside. Following this, comfort was considered as a response to suffering, recognising that different types of communication via hands, eyes and voice would be needed depending on how the person was managing their suffering. Finally, how carers could develop understanding and how to relate to people experiencing suffering was discussed, including an exploration of intuition.

Further study

The Well-being Institute on the Cambridge University website offers a wide range of information and resources that are evidence based. It also explores policy and personal development. The institute puts on events and you can subscribe to a news section. See: www.wellbeing.group.cam.ac.uk/

References

Barker, S. (2007) *Vital Notes for Nurses: Psychology*. Oxford: Blackwell.

Barker, S. (2011) *Midwives' Emotional Care of Women Becoming Mothers*. Newcastle upon Tyne: Cambridge Scholars Publishing.

Barker, S. (2013) *Nursing Care of Older People*. London: Learning Matters/Sage.

Bauman, B. (1961) 'Diversities in conceptions of health and fitness', *Journal of Health and Human Behavior*, 2: 39–46.

Benner, P. (1984) *From Novice to Expert: Excellence and Power in Clinical Nursing Practice*. Menlo Park, CA: Addison-Wesley.

Benner, P. and Wrubel, J. (1989) *The Primacy of Caring: Stress and Coping in Health and Illness*. Menlo Park, CA: Addison-Wesley.

Benner, P., Stutphen, M., Leonard, V., Day, L. and Shulman, L. (2010) *Educating Nurses: A Call for Radical Transformation*. Chichester: Wiley and Sons

Bentham, J. (1988) *The Principles of Morals and Legislation*. New York: Prometheus Books.

Blaxter, M. (1990) *Health and Lifestyles*. London: Routledge.

Carper, B.A. (1978) 'Fundamental patterns of knowing in nursing', *Advances in Nursing Science*, 1 (1): 13–24.

Davies, J. (2011) 'Positive and negative models of suffering: An anthropology of our shifting cultural consciousness of emotional discontent', *Anthropology of Consciousness*, 22 (2): 188–200.

Davis-Floyd, R. and Davis, E. (1996) 'Intuition as authoritative knowledge in midwifery and home births', *Medical Anthropology Quarterly*, 10 (2): 237–69.

Department of Health (DH) (2007) *Department of Health Commissioning Framework for Health and Wellbeing*. Available at: www.rcpa.org.uk/MyFiles/Files/Mar07-DoHCommissioning Framework for Health and Wellbeing.pdf (accessed June 2015).

Eriksson, J. (2014) 'Freud's psychoanalysis: A moral cure', *International Journal of Psychoanalysis*, 95: 663–75.

Frankl, V. (1963) *Man's Search for Meaning*, 3rd edn. New York: Simon and Schuster.

Goleman, D. (1998) *Working with Emotional Intelligence*. New York, NY: Bantum Books.

Goleman, D. (2004) *Emotional Intelligence and Working with Emotional Intelligence*. London: Bloomsbury.

Harris, I. (2007) 'The gift of suffering', in N.E. Johnston and A. Scholler-Jaquish (eds), *Meaning in Suffering: Caring Practices in Health Professions*. Madison, WI: University of Wisconsin Press, pp. 60–97.

Hildingsson, I. and Häggström, T. (1999) 'Midwives' lived experiences of being supportive to prospective mothers/parents during pregnancy', *Midwifery*, 15: 82–91.

Johns, C. (1995) 'Framing learning through reflection within Carper's fundamental ways of knowing in nursing', *Journal of Advanced Nursing*, 22 (2): 226-234

Johns, C. (2000) *Becoming a Reflective Practitioner*. Oxford: Blackwell Science.

Johns, C. (2013) *Becoming a Reflective Practitioner*, 4th edn. Oxford: Wiley-Blackwell.

Johnston, E. (2013) 'Strengthening a praxis of suffering: Teaching-learning practices', *Nursing Science Quarterly*, 26 (3): 230–5.

Kitwood, T. (1997) *Dementia Reconsidered: The Person Comes First*. Buckingham: Open University Press.

Kitwood, T. and Bredin, K. (1992) 'Towards a theory of dementia care: Personhood and well-being', *Ageing and Society*, 12 (3): 269–87.

The Lancet (2009) 'What is health? The ability to adapt', 373 (9666): 781. Available at: www.thelancet.com/journals/lancet/article/PIIS0140673609604566/fulltext?rss=yes (accessed June 2015).

Milton, C.L. (2013) 'Suffering', *Nursing Science Quarterly*, 26 (3): 226–8.

Morrison, V. and Bennett, P. (2012) *Introduction to Health Psychology*, 3rd edn. Harlow: Pearson.

Morse, J.M. (2000) 'Responding to the cues of suffering', *Health Care for Women International*, 21: 1–9.

Morse, J.M. (2001) 'Towards a praxis theory of suffering', *Advances in Nursing Science*, 24 (1): 47–59.

Morse, J.M., Bottorff, J., Anderson, G., O'Brien, B. and Solberg, S. (1992) 'Beyond empathy: Expanding expressions of caring', *Journal of Advanced Nursing*, 17: 809–21.

Morse, J.M., Bottorff, J.L. and Hutchinson, S. (1994) 'The phenomenology of comfort', *Journal of Advanced Nursing*, 20: 189–95.

Morse, J.M., Bottorff, J.L. and Hutchinson, S. (1995) 'The paradox of comfort', *Nursing Research*, 44 (1): 14–19.

NHS Careers (2015) *Health Psychologists*. Available at: www.nhscareers.nhs.uk/explore-by-career/psychological-therapies/careers-in-psychological-therapies/psychologist/health-psychologist/ (accessed June 2015).

Ólafsdóttir, Ó.Á. (2009) 'Inner knowing and emotions in the midwife–woman relationship', in B. Hunter and R. Deery (eds), *Emotions in Midwifery and Reproduction*. Basingstoke: Palgrave Macmillan, pp. 192–210.

Parse, R.R. (2010) 'Human dignity: A humanbecoming ethical phenomenon', *Nursing Science Quarterly*, 22: 305–9.

Polkinghorne, D.E. (2004) *Practice and the Human Sciences: The Case for a Judgement-Based Practice of Care*. New York: State University of New York, pp. 129–50.

Public Health England (2014) *Global Health Strategy 2014–2019*. Available at: www.gov.uk/government/uploads/system/uploads/attachment_data/file/354156/Global_Health_Strategy_final_version_for_publication_12_09_14.pdf (accessed June 2015).

Rehnsfeldt, A. and Eriksson, K. (2004) 'The progression of suffering implies alleviated suffering', *Scandinavian Journal Caring Science*, 18: 26472.

Schuiling, K.D. and Sampselle, C.M. (1999) 'Comfort in labor and midwifery art', *Image: Journal of Nursing Scholarship*, 31 (1): 77–81.

Schulz, R., Herbert, R.S., Dew, M.A., Brown, S.L., Scheier, M.F., Beach, S.R., Czaja, S.J., Martire, L.M., Coon, D., Langa, K.M., Gitlin, L.N., Stevens, S.B. and Nichols, L. (2007) 'Patient suffering and caregiver compassion: New opportunities for research, practice, and policy', *Gerontology*, 47 (1): 4–13.

Social Care Institute of Excellence (SCIE) (2005) *Independence, Wellbeing and Choice*. Available at: www.scie.org.uk/publications/consultation/adultgreenpaper.pdf (accessed June 2015).

Todres, L. (2008) 'Being with that: The relevance of embodied understanding for practice', *Qualitative Health Research*, 18 (11): 1566–73.

Todres, L., Galvin, K.T. and Holloway, I. (2009) 'The humanization of healthcare: A value framework for qualitative research', *International Journal of Qualitative Studies on Health and Wellbeing*, 4 (2): 68–77.

World Health Organization (WHO) (1948) 'Preamble to the Constitution of the World Health Organization as Adopted by the International Health Conference, New York, 19–22 June, 1946; Signed on 22 July 1946 by the Representatives of 61 States. (*Official Records of the World Health Organization*, No. 2, p. 100) and entered into force on 7 April 1948.

WHO (1986) *Ottawa Charter for Health Promotion*. Available at: www.who.int/healthpromotion/conferences/previous/ottawa/en/ (accessed June 2015).

4 Compassionate Care

Janet Scammell

> The NHS belongs to the people … It touches our lives at times of basic human need, when care and compassion are what matter most.
>
> *The NHS Constitution* (DH, 2015: 2)

Learning objectives

This chapter will explore the concepts of compassionate care and its context in contemporary practice. It will consider the understanding that psychology and its underpinning philosophies can offer to develop an understanding of this concept as experienced by health and social care practitioners. This chapter's learning objectives are to:

- Define and describe care, compassionate care and care culture
- Explore the context of contemporary care and why compassionate care is necessary
- Discuss models of care that may support compassionate care

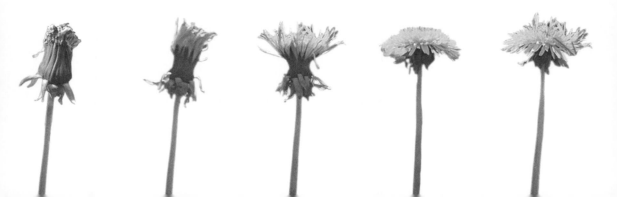

Activity 4.1   Critical thinking

Think of a time when you were offered compassionate care or offered compassionate care to someone else. Make a few notes about what this looked and felt like.

There is an outline answer at the end of the chapter.

Introduction

There have been emerging concerns about the quality of care being provided, especially to those most vulnerable within our society. Compassionate care is the current conception of high-quality care, and whilst there are problems with its definition, traditional models of care as well as the more contemporary ones can all help guide care practitioners. This chapter starts with exploring the contemporary context of care, progressing to an exploration of what care, particularly compassionate care, is and the culture within which this is provided. Traditional models of care will be explored and compared with more contemporary models of compassionate, humanised care. The chapter will end with an overview of the evidence base for the need for this type of care.

Contemporary impetus for compassionate care

The UK along with a number of other resource-rich countries is very fortunate in providing a health service that is free to all the population at the point of access. Founded in 1948, the NHS was highly influenced by the biomedical model of care, amongst great optimism that medical science would find technical solutions for most disease. Healthcare in many respects is very different today; we have successfully eradicated some major diseases and developed life-saving surgeries and medicines to prolong life. However, this has increased the number of people coping with multiple conditions, including those with chronic and complex illness living into very old age (DH, 2010). The need for healthcare, far from going down as envisaged at the onset of the NHS, has increased and with it the costs of care (Alderwick et al., 2015). The influence of business models has made care more technical and target driven; a diversity of private and public care providers have emerged and episodes of care are packaged to enable costing. Whereas in 1948 doctors were 'in charge' and patients passively complied with their instructions, as did other health workers, we now live in a consumer-led society, with clear legislation to support equal rights (Equality Act, 2010). Healthcare consumers now expect knowledgeable and competent healthcare practitioners, who involve them in care decisions, as well as efficient but compassionate care.

Service user movement

The terms 'service user' and 'carers' have become common in health and social care in the UK over the last decade. According to the SCIE (2015), these can be defined as people who are current or past users of services as well as potential users of services.

Carers are those people who are identified as supporting service users in some manner. Comprehensive involvement in the NHS by the public and service users from all
population groups has become a central plank of UK Government policy (DH, 2008).
Lakeman et al. (2007) write that the service user social movement started in the
1960s in an attempt to secure improved human rights and equality for marginalised
groups, notably people with mental illness, and led to huge service reform and more
humane treatment. The movement has in recent years spread to include all groups.
NHS strategy thus supports service user involvement in service development as well
as delivery:

> people want a greater degree of control and influence over their health and health-
> care. If anything, this is even more important for those who for a variety of reasons
> find it harder to seek out services or make themselves heard. (DH, 2008: 9)

The service user movement has profoundly influenced the current shape of health and
social care service provision. NHS strategy (DH, 2010) pledges to 'put patients and the
public first' and makes several important commitments to make this happen:

- Shared decision-making: No decision about me without me
- Patient access to information, to make choices about their care
- Patients will have choice of care provider
- Patients will be able to rate hospitals/departments according to care quality
- The system will focus on personalised care that reflects individuals' health and care
  needs, supports carers and encourages strong joint partnerships
- The collective voice of patients and the public will be strengthened at local and
  national levels

Media reports and official inquiries

The service user movement seems to have been successful in raising the profile of their
perspective within health and social care. However, despite this, there have been a series
of high-profile media scandals about poor care leading to a number of important official
inquiries. Two common themes are apparent: the client groups affected appear to be
some of the most vulnerable in society and unsafe and incompetent care was highlighted, including a lack of compassion.

The report *Death by Indifference* (MENCAP, 2007) set out the case for institutional
discrimination within the NHS for people with a learning disability. Through a series of
real case studies, the report highlights unequal access to care, physical health inequali-
ties, discrimination in terms of access to the full range of treatments (leading to unnecessary deaths) and a lack skills and knowledge of healthcare staff about the needs of this
client group and their carers. MENCAP argued that the Government response was
delayed and weak and claimed that they 'failed to place equal value on the lives of people
with a learning disability' (MENCAP, 2013).

Further scandal of abusive care of people with a learning disability uncovered by
secret filming at Winterbourne View Hospital shocked public and professionals alike.
Vulnerable clients were treated in a very dehumanised manner by care staff and most
distressing was the fact that this appeared to be viewed as 'normal' practice within that

culture. The subsequent Serious Case Review (Flynn, 2012) made many recommendations around the policies and procedures for safeguarding vulnerable adults, the need to strengthen 'whistleblowing' procedures for staff and others, and the requirement to review quality inspection and commissioning systems.

Around the same time, care quality in relation to another group of vulnerable adults was also causing concerns. The Parliamentary and Health Service Ombudsman (2011) produced a report into the care of 10 older people. Following a rising tide of complaints about care, the Ombudsman initiated this investigation and found unnecessary suffering, pain and indignity whilst in NHS care, resulting in the deterioration of their health status. Most damning perhaps is the comment:

> The investigations reveal an attitude – both personal and institutional – which fails to recognise the humanity and individuality of the people concerned and to respond to them with sensitivity, compassion and professionalism. (Parliamentary and Health Service Ombudsman, 2011: 7)

This indicated a clear gap between the espoused values and principles of the NHS and the health professions, and the reality of practice.

Unfortunately, similar findings were to emerge from an extensive Public Inquiry lasting over two years into failings in care in the Mid Staffordshire NHS Foundation Trust. The executive summary (Francis, 2013) catalogued 'appalling conditions of care' that were allowed to 'flourish' over a period of three years in the main hospital serving Stafford and district. Not only did the hospital culture allow poor care to become normalised, but also the internal and external quality procedures did not identify warning signs to indicate any cause for concern. In fact, it was the efforts of patients' relatives and staff whistleblowers that finally prompted the investigation. The report concluded that:

> the system as a whole failed in its most essential duty – to protect patients from unacceptable risks of harm and from unacceptable, and in some cases inhumane, treatment that should never be tolerated in any hospital. (Francis, 2013: 8)

In total, 290 recommendations for improvement were made targeted at all levels, including the Department of Health, healthcare professions' regulatory bodies, external quality assurance agencies, Trust Boards and governing bodies, medical education and training providers, clinical leaders and individual practitioners. The fallout has been significant and will be discussed further, but for the purpose of this chapter it is useful to reflect on how those in the care business failed to care in a compassionate, humanised way.

Similar failings in care in the Maternity Unit of Furness General Hospital were uncovered following another official investigation (Kirkup, 2015). The report revealed a long-term highly dysfunctional maternity unit, with poor leadership and team working, substandard competence and inadequate regulation and quality monitoring. This noxious culture led to maternal and infant deaths and again, like in Stafford, patient and relative concerns were ignored and external quality assurance mechanisms failed to identify and act upon concerns.

Department of Health policy

It is clear from these reports that failures and specifically a lack of compassion in care were not only system-wide but also at an individual level. Whilst it is tempting to think that 'one bad apple ruined the barrel', given the extent of the problems uncovered, it would seem that non-compassionate care was allowed to become the norm. In other words, even if my care is good, is it compassionate if I ignore poor care which I observe? Under pressure to address these concerns and in response to the Francis report, the DH took action and one month later published their response *Patients First and Foremost* (DH, 2013). In the foreword by the Secretary of State for Health, he notes that:

> A toxic culture was allowed to develop unchecked which fostered the normalisation of cruelty and the victimisation of those brave enough to speak up. (DH, 2013: 5)

A Statement of Common Purpose signed by representatives of government, professional regulators and quality assurance agencies is outlined and includes a renewed commitment to the values of the NHS set out in the Constitution (DH, 2015), one of which is the commitment to compassion in care:

> We ensure that compassion is central to the care we provide and respond with humanity and kindness to each person's pain, distress, anxiety or need. We search for the things we can do, however small, to give comfort and relieve suffering. We find time for patients, their families and carers, as well as those we work alongside. We do not wait to be asked, because we care. (DH, 2013: 9)

This commitment is important because it could be argued that measurable, technical care tasks tends to be 'rewarded' over compassionate care and hence the latter is not valued in practice.

NHS England's *Compassion in Practice*: The 6Cs

In support of this commitment at policy level, the Chief Nursing Officer for England, Jane Cummings, published her vision and strategy for Nursing, Midwifery and Care Staff *Compassion in Practice* (DH, 2012) as a way of raising the profile of key values from the NHS Constitution that must underpin practice. Commonly known as the 6Cs (see Table 4.1), this strategy focuses on developing a culture of compassionate caregiving through promoting appropriate attitudes and behaviours from the professional caregivers:

> As our NHS helps people to live longer, care needs are changing, and our health and care services are evolving to meet these needs. What hasn't changed is the fundamental human need to be looked after with *care* and *compassion*, by a professional who is *competent* and *communicates* well, by someone with the *courage* to make changes that improve people's care and deliver the best and the *commitment* to deliver this all day, every day [emboldened words are from the original paper]. (DH, 2012: 5)

Table 4.1   *Compassion in Practice* (DH, 2012: 13): the 6Cs

1.	Care	Care is our core business and that of our organisations and the care we deliver helps the individual person and improves the health of the whole community. Caring defines us and our work. People receiving care expect it to be right for them consistently throughout every stage of their life.
2.	Compassion	Compassion is how care is given through relationships based on empathy, respect and dignity. It can also be described as intelligent kindness and is central to how people perceive their care.
3.	Competence	Competence means all those in caring roles must have the ability to understand an individual's health and social needs. It is also about having the expertise, clinical and technical knowledge to deliver effective care and treatments based on research and evidence.
4.	Communication	Communication is central to successful caring relationships and to effective team working. Listening is as important as what we say and do. It is essential for 'No decision about me without me'. Communication is the key to a good workplace with benefits for those in our care and staff alike.
5.	Courage	Courage enables us to do the right thing for the people we care for, to speak up when we have concerns. It means we have the personal strength and vision to innovate and to embrace new ways of working.
6.	Commitment	A commitment to our patients and populations is a cornerstone of what we do. We need to build on our commitment to improve the care and experience of our patients. We need to take action to make this vision and strategy a reality for all and meet the health and social care challenges ahead.

Case study

 Jack and Sue

Jack is an elderly, retired man with type 2 diabetes who lives on his own in a rural area. He is no longer able to mobilise independently. A call from Jack's care agency requested an urgent nurse visit from a district nurse due to a suspected ulcer on his foot. On arrival and entering Jack's room it was evident that he was bed bound. After removing Jack's socks, an offensive odour was apparent and on examination he had a severe infected ulcer on his foot. Before cleaning and dressing the wound the district nurse Sue contacted the surgery for advice, as she was quite concerned about the severity and progression of the ulcer. The triage doctor agreed to visit to assess the wound. On arrival, the doctor introduced himself to Sue, completely ignoring myself (a nursing student) and Jack, and examined his foot, whilst asking Sue about Jack's general health. The nurse recognised Jack, was being ignored and addressed the same questions to Jack. Following the examination, Sue asked to speak to the doctor outside of the room before he left. She explained that Jack had full mental capacity and was able to answer for himself, and she felt that the doctor rushed the consultation. The doctor did not apologise to Sue or Jack and left without saying goodbye.

Case study provided by Amelia Payne

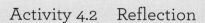

Activity 4.2 Reflection

Take a few minutes to reflect on this case study. What would you have done in this situation?

As this is a reflection, there is no outline answer at the end of the chapter.

Sue visited Jack to assess his needs and went on to provide appropriate *care* based on that assessment. With Jack's best interest in mind, she was aware of the limits of her *competence* and called for medical advice concerning the infected wound. Sue demonstrated *compassion* towards Jack when he was ignored by the doctor and treated him with respect by *communicating* with him directly. She demonstrated *courage* by challenging the doctor about his communication and rushed consultation, upholding a *commitment* to the values of her profession and the NHS.

Response of regulatory bodies for health and social care professionals

As a result of these reports criticising publicly funded care, the organisations that regulate health and social care professionals were tasked by Government to review their professional and ethical codes of practice.

The Health and Care Professions Council (HCPC) regulates health, psychological and social work professionals' standards of conduct, performance and ethics. Their code, last reviewed in 2008, does not specifically mention compassion, but indicates a commitment to this concept. The code states that:

> You must treat service users with respect and dignity. If you are providing care, you must work in partnership with your service users and involve them in their care as appropriate. (HCPC, 2008: 8)

The General Medical Council (GMC) is like the other regulators – an independent organisation that exists to protect patients, and specifically to improve medical education and regulate practice. The GMC reviewed their Standards and Ethics Guidance for Doctors and associated guide *Good Medical Practice* (GMC, 2013) after the publication of the final Francis report. The word 'compassion' is not mentioned, but in the section on the 'Duties of a doctor', it states that they are expected to 'Take prompt action if you think that a patient's safety, dignity or comfort is being compromised' as well as 'Treat patients as individuals and respect their dignity'.

The Nursing and Midwifery Council (NMC) also exists to protect the public, setting standards for education and conduct. Their code was extensively reviewed in light of the Francis report. The NMC professional standards of practice and behaviour for nurses and midwives (2015), refers to compassion four times. Practitioners are expected to:

> Treat people as individuals and uphold their dignity: To achieve this, you must:
>
> 1.1 treat people with kindness, respect and compassion

2.6   recognise when people are anxious or in distress and respond compassionately and politely.

3.2   recognise and respond compassionately to the needs of those who are in the last few days and hours of life

11.2   make sure that everyone you delegate tasks to is adequately supervised and supported so they can provide safe and compassionate care.

It can be seen from this brief review of professional codes that compassion is a key value that should underpin practice as well as professional education. Making this a reality is the focus of the rest of the chapter.

Duty of candour

Francis (2013) argued that NHS culture did not support 'whistleblowing' (Figure 4.1) and advocated that the mechanisms to support this were essential to ensure compassionate care. He states that at the heart of the failures in Mid Staffordshire Hospital was a lack of openness, transparency and candour in the information about care produced by the Trust and that their version of events was not questioned by those tasked to quality-assure care. Francis felt that this lack of candour operated at all levels because if staff had been honest, open and truthful in what they observed, this may have prevented the failure to uphold fundamental care standards. In response the NMC and GMC worked together to develop clearer guidance for practitioners about what was meant by candour in professional practice and how this would be enacted. Following wide consultation, new guidance on the professional duty of candour was published (GMC and NMC, 2015). The personal duty of candour tasks practitioners to be honest with patients when things go wrong and to take appropriate actions. However, there is also an organisational duty to develop a culture where openness and honesty are the norm and part of a learning culture.

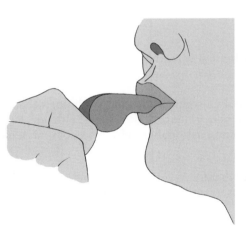

Figure 4.1   Whistleblowing

In publishing this guidance, the regulators are perhaps recognising the power dynamics within care cultures and the need to empower individuals to 'do the right thing' within that culture, hopefully thereby affecting change from within. Mistakes happen but health professions must own up to these and seek to learn from them personally and within organisations to prevent similar events happening to others.

Culture of care

The word 'care' can be used in a number of ways: it can refer to both personal characteristics and overt behaviours; it can be a noun or a verb. Indeed, when linked to other words, it can become a vast number of social concepts, organisations or philosophy, for example social care, child care, care ethics or duty of care. Despite this ambiguity, most people feel they have a sense of what 'care is' and what 'to be caring' means. To provide a precise definition is far from easy. For many professions, particularly caring professions, to develop a sound understanding of the term is, however, necessary.

Problems with definition and clarification can be seen in the Nursing and Midwifery Council's (NMC, 2004: 13) leaflet, provided with the code of professional conduct for nurses and midwives. It offered 'provide help or comfort' as a definition of care, whereas the recently updated code does not provide a short definition at all. The NMC 2015 code of conduct, whilst not providing a concise definition, does provide clear standards on how to demonstrate care. The General Medical Council (GMC, 2015) states that the first priority of the doctor is to 'care for their patients', whilst the Health and Care Professions Council (HCPC, 2008) in their standards do not refer to care; they make statements related to 'support' and 'help' in a similar way to the NMC.

To support the person starting a caring career there are many introductory texts that offer an explanation of the concept of care and caring. They suggest that there are a number of factors that constitute this term. These include elements such as time, place of care, needs of all those involved (both caregiver and receiver), alongside skills, knowledge and attitudes. The skills and attitudes that should be demonstrated are sensitivity and understanding as well as the ability to support the person or help fulfil their needs. The caregiver will need good communication skills, including empathy and self-awareness. It can clearly be seen from this description that caring is a complex and skilful task. There is, though, a widely held assumption that these skills are innate and do not require learning and hence do not attract the reward or status that might be expected (Bolton, 2000; John and Parsons, 2006).

Whilst care and caring are recognised as an essential component in all the helping professions (Morrison, 1992) and there is a general sense of a shared meaning of the term by the public, the concept of a culture of care is a more contentious issue. This has been a particular area for concern in England and Wales over the last few years. One definition of culture is given as follows:

> Culture is socially determined and shapes many aspects of our identity, including our beliefs, values and behaviour. It encompasses many factors, including race, ethnicity, religion, gender, sexuality, age, generation, class, life experience and lifestyle. (Thurgood, 2009: 630)

Culture has been described as the 'lens' through which the world can be seen. It includes a set of assumptions about the world which may be expressed **symbolically** through language, art and ritual; culture is our worldview (Draper and McSherry, 2007).

Napoles et al. (2010: 390) offer a consensual definition of culture; they write:

> A consensual definition of culture found in the literature is that it consists of shared group behaviours and norms, such as traditions, values, beliefs, attitudes, symbols, language, religion and social roles of an **ethnic** group.

This can be interpreted as culture being the shared meanings of a distinct group of people use to manage their everyday experiences. Kitwood (1997), whose theory was explored in Chapter 3, offers a similar definition. He stated that culture is the patterns of behaviour that give meaning to experiences and provide structure for group actions and interactions. Culture can be experienced **explicitly** or **implicitly**; we are able to be consciously aware of our culture, and that of others, but it can also influence us at an unconscious level. There are considered to be three main elements of culture: its knowledge or **power base**, behavioural norms and an **ideology** or belief system. Kitwood identified, through his research into dementia care cultures, that dominant cultures are difficult to change. Throughout this book, the knowledge or power base of caring is being explored alongside the explicit behaviours seen, but it will be useful to examine ideologies here to facilitate understanding of the care culture.

Compassion

Activity 4.3   Creative thinking

Consider your notes from Activity 4.1; how would you define compassion?

There is an outline answer at the end of the chapter.

As with care, 'compassion' is a difficult word to define despite a general belief that everyone knows what it is when it occurs. Recognition of compassion may have similarities to comfort as it is most noticed when it is not being experienced. A common understanding of compassion is that it is the demonstration of warmth, kindness and generosity, whereas a more literal definition would be that it is the suffering of one person with another.

Stickley and Spandler (2014) encourage us to recognise the link between compassion and empathy; they discuss compassion 'in action'. Accepting this link, the NMC (2009) inform us compassion is about recognising how the person feels, to be empathetic but also to have the desire to care for them to improve their experience. It is 'how care is given through relationships based on empathy, respect and dignity' (DH and NHS Commissioning Board, 2012: 13), whereas Goetz et al. (2010: 351) define compassion as 'a distinct affective experience whose primary function is to facilitate cooperation and protection of the weak and those who suffer'. This highlights the experience of emotion, a personal feeling response to the other's suffering (perhaps empathy), and the motivation to help others.

Likewise Buddhists, who believe that to live is to suffer, identify compassion as the motivation to relieve the suffering in others but they do not suggest it involves an emotional experience (Brazier, 2003). In this sense, the person has the interpersonal intention and motivation to relieve distress but this can be undertaken without a personal emotional experience.

Gilbert (2009) recognises compassion in an evolutionary sense identifying the role of threat, motivation and soothing systems. His model provides an explanation of the use of compassion through an appraisal process. As with Buddhists, Gilbert understands compassion as a concept of motivation. He provides a personal intention, a personal reward, whereas Buddhists focus on the interpersonal intention and not on personal benefit. Gilbert's ideas are discussed in more detail later in the chapter. Both Gilbert and

Buddhists recognise that compassion involves action; it is the motivation to action but also includes the resulting behaviour.

We can see that for all of these authors compassion is about the motivation to alleviate another's suffering whether that is due to personal emotional engagement with them (empathy) or spiritual beliefs.

Models of care

The term 'models of care' refers to the overarching approach and principles by which care is organised. The model can be at the level of organisations, for example a hospital adopting the Watson (2007) approach, or at the level of a profession, with psychotherapists adopting the Gilbert (2009) approach. Many models of care have evolved for nursing but can be useful for a range of health practitioners.

Models are based on a philosophy of care influenced by a perspective or view on the way care recipients and caregivers are perceived. Prior to the Enlightenment, care was much influenced by theology; whilst this is less evident, it remains apparent in some current care models (Roach, 1987; Eriksson, 2002). However, modern medicine is influenced by the biomedical model whereby thinking and explaining about disease is based on biological factors (Barry and Yuill, 2008):

- The body is viewed as separate to the mind
- The body is likened to a machine that needs repairing
- Emphasis is on technological means to 'fix' problems
- Physical reasons for disease tend to be prioritised over psychological and social ones
- All diseases have a known aetiology or cause (although we may not know what this is as yet)

Whilst this is a very successful model in many respects, it values curing activities over caring activities, with profound implications for the way care is organised and the status of those providing it. Cure is the aim and so where cure is possible these specialities have a high status and so do the people associated with them, both healthcare professionals and the clients themselves. Biomedicine is particularly effective in acute situations where the cause of illness can be located through clear symptoms that can be linked to a diagnosis and then treated, for example a patient with a broken leg. It is less effective in situations of multiple pathology and chronic illness. Other models of care have evolved alongside biomedicine to focus on the needs of the wider range of patients and care, as well as to reflect roles allied to medicine such as nurses, midwives and other health professionals.

Florence Nightingale, 1820–1910

One of the most famous nurses in recent history is Florence Nightingale. As a woman born into upper-class Victorian society in England, she was an unlikely candidate to influence nursing, as at the time it was far from being perceived as a respectable occupation. However, she was moved by reports of poor care for wounded British soldiers fighting in the Crimean War (1854–56) and used her impressive organisational abilities and knowledge of statistics and scientific methods to radically improve this situation. Her Christian beliefs shaped her sense of moral duty that 'something had to be done' and she used her social and political connections to train and send a group of 'suitable' middle-class ladies out to the Crimea to set up and run a military hospital. Cleanliness and care greatly improved and her approach profoundly influenced the early foundations of professional nurse education in the UK.

Nightingale wrote *Notes on Nursing* (1859) and whilst not identified as a model of care, it was in fact just that, as it outlined simple health rules that were not familiar at the time such as the importance of cleanliness, nourishment, natural light, sleep and a peaceful environment in influencing well-being and promoting recovery. Influenced by Christian ideology, Nightingale also had much to say about the good character of a nurse: they should be selfless and strive to relieve suffering through acts of compassion (Nightingale, 1859). Her impact was profound as this still reflects society's perception and expectations of nurses and nursing today.

Madeleine Leininger, 1925–2012

Leininger was a nursing theorist from the USA who proposed a cultural theory of care. Her theory, *Cultural Care Diversity and Universality* (1991, cited Leininger and McFarland 2006), highlighted the growing trend of globalisation and its impact on healthcare; when people from diverse cultures encounter one another for the first time, there is a possibility that ethnocentric attitudes negatively impact on the care relationship. As with other care theorists (Eriksson, 2002; Watson, 2007), Leininger conceived care as a humanistic and scientific endeavour that was essential for human growth and sense of well-being. She stated that there cannot be any 'cure' without 'care' and that care occurs within a culture of care. She accepted and acknowledged that cultures differ (diversity) but argues that they also have commonalities (universality). Leininger recognises that culture is embedded within our worldview; in other words our culture influences the way we perceive the world around us and this in turn affects the way we behave. Thus, culture is **ethnohistorical** (cultural development over time), influenced by social structures and environmental contexts.

Leininger's model recognises that care cultures have **emic** and **etic** features; they have **generic** and professional components. For care to be congruent and therapeutic, practitioners need to be aware of their and other people's care culture and their underpinning values, beliefs, expressions and patterns (life-ways). For example culture is often associated with faith systems. Faith influences the meaning we ascribe to illness, suffering and death. The practitioner may view these concepts differently from a care recipient from another culture. Compassionate care is facilitated by therapeutic relationships; knowledge and understanding of diversity enables the practitioner to build trust and this provides respectful, sensitive care.

Jean Watson, 1970s

Like Leininger, Watson (2007), in developing her theory of *Human Science and Human Care*, believed that medical 'cure' was reliant on 'care'. She advocates a holistic approach like other care theorists, arguing that a human being is 'greater than the sum of his or her parts'. Her focus is transpersonal caring; she argues that viewing the person as an illness rather than focusing on their holistic well-being will hinder recovery. The practitioner's role is to provide a caring environment that is accepting of the person and promotes growth. Watson identifies 10 carative factors (see Table 4.2); these can be seen to have strong spiritual influences, and are based on existential phenomenology and humanism (see Chapter 5), notably the theory of Rogers.

Table 4.2 Developed from Watson, 2007 and 2010

Ten carative factors (2007)	Ten carative processes (2010)
Formation of a humanistic-altruistic value systems	Practising loving-kindness and equanimity within context of caring consciousness
Instillation of faith-hope	Being authentically present and enabling, and sustaining the deep belief system and subjective life world of self and one-being-cared-for
Cultivation of sensitivity to self and others	Cultivating one's own spiritual practices and transpersonal self; going beyond ego self
Developing helping-trust relationships	Developing and sustaining a helping-trusting, authentic caring relationship
Assistance with gratification of human needs	Being present to and supportive of the expression of positive and negative feelings
Promotion and acceptance of the expression of positive and negative feelings	Creatively using self and all ways of knowing as part of the caring process; engaging in artistry of caring-healing practices
Systematic use of a creative problem-solving caring process for decision-making	Engaging in genuine teaching-learning experience that attends to wholeness and meaning, attempting to stay within other's frame of reference
Promotion of transpersonal teaching-learning	Creating healing environment at all levels, whereby wholeness, beauty, comfort, dignity and peace are potentiated
Provision for a supportive, protective and/or corrective mental, physical, societal and spiritual environment	Assisting with basic needs, with an intentional caring consciousness; administering 'human care essentials' which potentiate alignment of mind-body-spirit; wholeness in all aspects of care
Allowance for existential-phenomenological-spiritual forces	Opening and attending to mysterious dimensions of one's life-death; soul care for self and the one-being-cared for; 'allowing and being open to miracles'

There have been at least 40 studies conducted using Watson's theoretical framework, making it influential particularly in North America. Watson herself has also continued to develop her model of caring from the 10 carative factors; she has developed the 10 carative processes to guide care practice. These are expressed in more easily accessible terms but still may appear more aesthetic than practical. She goes further to develop these processes into practical actions that she calls 'Caritas Consciousness'.

Simone Roach, 1980s

Roach (1987) established her theory of human caring in nursing. She believes that caring is an intrinsic trait of human beings. This involves the capacity to care, 'calling forth' this capacity, in response to some internal or external motivation and displaying this in caring behaviours. Roach is clearly influenced by her Christian beliefs, as well as, like Watson, the philosophical approach of phenomenology, particularly Heideggerian hermeneutic phenomenology (see Chapter 5). Her model of caring outlines the attributes involved (what the practitioner does when caring), which she terms the 'six Cs': compassion, competence, confidence, conscience, comportment and commitment. Her work clearly influenced the development of the key components of the NHS nursing and midwifery strategy in the UK.

Case study

Matt and Ruby

A 17-year-old boy called Matt was brought into the operating theatre where I was on a clinical placement. He lived with his foster mother Ruby. He had a learning disability and was very agitated. The theatre staff allowed Ruby to come into theatre to reassure Matt and keep him calm. Normally, a patient of this age would not be allowed a parent/carer to be with them, but the staff tailored care to his needs. Matt's foster mother calmed him down by comparing what was happening to *Holby City* (a TV soap) and the theatre staff were able to join in. This really helped to change the 'atmosphere' for Matt, and the operation was able to go ahead as planned.

Case study from Imogen Fox

The theatre staff showed *compassion* by imagining the situation from Matt's perspective and acknowledging his fears. They showed *commitment* to make care better and did this by inviting someone Matt knew to accompany him. This was influenced by *conscience*: their knowledge of the impact of unfamiliar situations on some people with moderate learning disabilities made them ensure that Matt did not suffer discrimination due to his condition. The staff wanted to deliver *competent* effective care but realised this depended on Matt's cooperation and so had to adapt their practice to facilitate this. They had the *confidence* to adapt protocols to suit his care needs and *comportment* to justify this decision.

Katie Eriksson, 2000s

Many of the models of care emanate from North America. In contrast Katie Eriksson is a Scandinavian academic who developed a theory of caritative caring. The caritative principle is one found in Christianity but reflected in a number of other world religions, meaning 'charitable in nature'. It is linked with the notions of serving and love for other. In Scandinavian countries, programmes for health professions are not based in faculties of biological science or medical science (reflecting a biomedical approach) but in faculties of caring sciences, which reflects a more humanistic orientation to health professional education. Outlining her theory (Eriksson, 2002), she argued that caring science was on the cusp of change; in response to the dominance of technology in care, Eriksson, like others (Galvin and Todres, 2013; Watson, 2007), argues for a more humanistic orientation. The influence of hermeneutical phenomenology is evident in her work as she advocates a focus on the nature of being (or the ontological core of practice) to empathetically respond to patients' care needs in an increasingly complex healthcare environment. Eriksson's phenomenon of caring is informed by eight basic assumptions:

- The human being is fundamentally an entity of body, soul and spirit
- The human being is fundamentally a religious being, but all human beings have not recognised this dimension
- The human being is fundamentally holy. Human dignity means accepting the human obligation of serving with love, of existing for the sake of others
- Health means a movement in becoming, being and doing, and striving for integrity and holiness which is compatible with bearable suffering

- The basic category of caring is suffering
- The basic motive of caring is the *caritas* motive
- Caring implies alleviating suffering in charity, love, faith and hope. Natural basic caring is expressed through tending, playing and teaching in a sustained caring relationship
- Caring relationship offers the context of caring, the caritative ethic developed from the ethos of love, responsibility and sacrifice.

A caring relationship forms the meaningful context of caring and derives its origin from the ethos of love, responsibility and sacrifice, that is, a caritative ethic (Eriksson, 2002: 62).

This approach, whilst clearly informed by ethical principles to guide practice, differs in that it is founded on the notion that the underpinning motivation of the carer is love and charity or *caritas*; this approach, Eriksson argues, leads to care that respects human dignity.

Kendrick and Robinson, 2000s

Finally in this section, another model clearly influenced by theological perspectives is termed 'loving care' or 'moderated love' (Kendrick and Robinson, 2002). Other theorists in nursing (Freshwater and Stickley, 2004) and midwifery (Hall, 2001) have suggested that the caring relationship is a type of loving relationship. Kendrick and Robinson (2002: 292) state that 'tender loving care' (TLC) reflects the core purpose of nurse–patient engagement, through 'beneficent attending' to sustain vulnerable individuals. The motivation they argue is compassion towards a stranger to make an empathetic connection to be with them in their suffering. Interestingly, the abbreviation TLC is frequently used by practitioners in situations where no cure is possible, death is imminent and comfort is the major aim; it is less common in general care and some may consider the notion of loving relationships as too intimate or close. However, Kendrick and Robinson (2002) write that this type of love would be recognised as *agape*, as accepted within the Christian tradition, and the **relational ethic** applied, where ethical action is situated in the relationship or commitment to one another.

Contemporary compassionate care frameworks

As has been discussed above, the impetus for compassionate care in the UK has been driven in recent years by a number of high-profile scandals concerning care quality. This has not only influenced policy and regulation but also brought to the fore the value of care frameworks as guides for practitioners. Some recent developments are now explored.

The BOND framework of compassionate care: Baughan and Smith (2013)

Baughan and Smith (2013) developed a framework that unpacks the contemporary nature of compassionate caring. Working from their analysis of stories of care from nursing students, registered practitioners and service users, they constructed a framework composed of 18 caring indicators; these are then categorised into four interrelated or 'bonded' themes which 'clarify and encapsulate what a caring nurse is and does' (p. 147). The first letter of each theme forms the apposite word 'BOND', hence the framework name (see Table 4.3).

Table 4.3 The BOND framework of compassionate care

Interrelated theme	Caring indicators
B = being and becoming	Being a caring presence
	Being empathetic
	Becoming more emotionally intelligent
	Being conscientious and ready to learn
	Being adaptable, flexible, creative
O = overcoming obstacles	Fostering resilience and capability
	Reframing the problem
	Maintaining non-discriminatory, non-judgemental practice
	Using preventative and restorative skills
	Working in effective partnerships
N = noticing	Systematic and holistic assessment
	The effects of cues and interactions
	Indicators of compassion fatigue
	The professional and ethical demands of caring
D = doing	Establishing therapeutic relationships
	Understanding and supporting informal carers
	Engaging in critical analysis and evaluation of practice
	Influencing the working environment

Source: Adapted from Baughan and Smith (2013: 138)

The framework is informed by concepts that underpin theory describing emotional intelligence (see Chapter 8), and highlights the fundamental need for practitioners to develop high levels of self-awareness in order to both work compassionately with service users and colleagues but also to **self-monitor** for signs of compassion fatigue. Whilst developed for nurses, the BOND framework provides a useful tool for other care professionals to develop our understanding of care interactions and in so doing influence how we deliver compassionate care.

Being and becoming theme

Baughan and Smith (2013) state that the way we care is closely tied to what we are like as people. We learn to 'be', that is, our beliefs and values shape who we are, but we also learn to 'become' as experiences change our perceptions about what is important in life. Both these aspects influence how we are perceived by others and highlight the importance of self-awareness in terms of understanding what we bring to caring interactions and situations. The caring indicator *being a caring presence* involves being sufficiently comfortable 'in our own skin' to be ready to connect with others and be available them. This is closely related with *being empathetic* and seeing service users as people first rather than diseased or disabled objects. In order to be effective, we need to *become more emotionally intelligent* to understand our emotional responses engendered by care scenarios and their impact. This means accepting the emotional labour associated with care work and *being conscientious and ready to learn more* to ensure our care is compassionate even in difficult situations. This may mean *being adaptable, flexible and creative* in trying to understand the lived experience of service users and make that compassionate connection.

Overcoming obstacles

This theme acknowledges the personal 'costs' associated with care work and considers the notion of resilience and strategies to enact it. Coping with adverse events and emotionally challenging situations on a long-term basis requires *fostering resilience and capability*; if we are unable to look after our own emotional health this is likely to compromise our ability to provide compassionate care. Working with an aggressive patient, for example, may leave us frustrated as we try to suppress our 'true' feelings; a more resilient response would be to *reframe the problem*, suspend our judgement of other people's behaviour, *maintain non-discriminatory practice* and view them as a vulnerable person with a health need. When we perceive people as 'problems' we can lose sight of the person and the opportunity to *use preventative and restorative skills* that could more positively reconnect the professional with the patient. *Working in effective partnerships* with patients and others in an authentic way is more likely to result in compassionate care (Figure 4.2).

Noticing

Imparting information is an important part of communication but so also is 'noticing' subtle cues and being aware of intuitive feelings, as this is aligned to our ability to offer

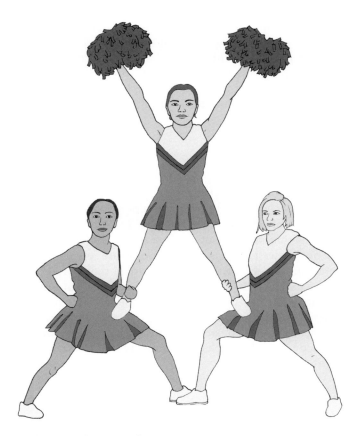

Figure 4.2   Partnership – working together

compassionate responses. With experience practitioners develop ever more refined *systematic and holistic assessment* skills which enable them to capture the obvious as well as notice more subtle signs to inform decision-making.

Case study

Mrs Perkins

Sometimes compassionate care can just be quantified in time spent with patients, not necessarily compassion within tasks. Time spent chatting with a patient can be precious and beneficial to a patient. I visited a Mrs Perkins to give some nursing care and could sense that she hadn't spoken to anyone in a while and wanted a chat. She insisted that I have a glass of ginger beer; usually, I would politely decline but clinical judgement suggested that this social interaction was important. So I sat and I chatted and listened and sipped my ginger beer. Yes, it took an extra 10 minutes of my time but it meant a lot to her. And if I am late [for the next visit] because someone feels more valued today, so be it.

Case study from Alex Oldham

Throughout the visit, the nurse is clearly assessing Mrs Perkins in a holistic sense and responding *to cues and interactions* to guide his decisions. If he felt stressed due to the pressure to get to the next visit, this would be an *indicator of compassion fatigue*, resulting in a far less compassionate interaction. Care would have been of an adequate quality but less humanised. Not only does Mrs Perkins feel valued, but the nurse also became conscious of Mrs Perkins' social isolation and could use this to inform further multidisciplinary care planning.

Doing

The last theme concerns demonstrating compassionate caring by doing, through practical skills and expertise. *Establishing therapeutic relationships* requires the development of trust at a deep or superficial level as this provides reassurance to the care recipient and enhances their sense of self-worth, as illustrated by the scenario with Mrs Perkins. Similarly, interventions that incorporate *understanding and supporting informal carers* are highly valued by service users as they demonstrate a valuing of their skills and knowledge in contributing to the compassionate care of their loved one. However, compassion must also be extended to ourselves as practitioners and nurtured in those we work with, as ultimately this will impact on care quality. We therefore need to routinely engage in *critical analysis and evaluation of practice* personally and in relation to our work culture. It is everyone's responsibility to monitor and *influence the working environment* for comprised practices which can ultimately lead to the 'toxic mix' highlighted in the Francis report (2013).

Compassion-focused therapy: Gilbert (2009)

Paul Gilbert is a clinical psychologist who describes the underpinning theory and process of applying a model of compassion to psychotherapy. Compassion-focused therapy is an integrated approach that draws upon evolutionary, social, developmental and Buddhist psychology and neuroscience. Gilbert observed that people with high levels of shame and self-criticism, often rooted in early trauma or abuse, experience difficulties in being kind to themselves or being self-compassionate. He hypothesised that in these individuals, the affect systems (regulating emotions) that help us to feel content and register human warmth are out of balance (Table 4.4). Rebalancing the systems is seen as one goal of compassion-focused therapy, with an emphasis on developing the social safeness/soothing system.

Table 4.4 Focus of behaviour related to emotion regulation

Emotion regulation system	Focus of behaviour
Threat and protection	Threat-focused
	Safety-seeking
Drive and excitement	Incentive/resource-focused
	Seeking and behaviour-activating
Contentment, soothing and social safeness	Affiliative-focused
	Soothing/safeness

Source: Adapted from Gilbert (2009)

Compassion-focused therapy revolves around compassionate mind training and this is attained through the therapist demonstrating the skills and attributes of compassion. The idea is that through the development of a compassionate relationship with the client, the therapist instils these skills to replace their self-critical and blaming stance. The therapist then helps the client to develop these compassionate attributes and skills and direct them towards self. This can be represented as an inner circle containing the attributes of compassion: sensitivity, empathy, distress tolerance, care for well-being, sympathy and non-judgement.

An outer ring represents the multimodal skills of compassion offered by the therapist, also common to other therapies: imagery, sensation, reasoning, behaviour, feeling and attention. These are offered in an overall environment of warmth, kindness and support. The focus of therapy is to generate and teach the client to self-generate an emotion towards self of self-warmth or self-kindness, or as Gilbert defines it, self-compassion. He argues that Buddhist psychology has a tradition of compassion-focused therapy but further outcome and process-focused research is required to demonstrate its efficacy (see Chapter 7).

Humanising Values Framework: Galvin and Todres (2013)

As healthcare has become more sophisticated, it has become more specialised and at times rather technical and task-focused (Galvin and Todres, 2013). The context of care delivery is also subject to increasing financial constraints in the UK and elsewhere, which may have led care to become somewhat target driven to enable measurement. Indeed the Francis report (2013) illustrated that a 'blind' focus on meeting targets, without perceiving and responding to the basic human needs of the person, results in poor-quality care. Observing these trends over the last decade, two philosophers and phenomenologists, Kathleen Galvin and Les Todres, made the stark comment that something significant seems to be missing in healthcare today and this seems to be an inattention to the 'things that make us feel more human' (Galvin and Todres, 2013: 1). Adopting a life world approach, they developed the Humanising Values Framework (HVF) which re-emphasises the values that should underpin authentic person-centred healthcare. Eight dimensions for humanising care are delineated, expressed as continua moving towards the polar opposite dimensions for dehumanising care. This approach has been applied to a number of clinical settings as well as professional education, and will be explored further in Chapter 5.

Compassionate relationship-centred care model: Dewar and Nolan (2013)

Much of the recent criticism of care that lacks compassion has concerned care for older people. Belinda Dewar's work is therefore very pertinent; she undertook an appreciative enquiry study which actively involved older people and their relatives as well as staff working in acute settings to develop and agree a definition of compassionate relationship-centred care. It is argued that care excellence depends on therapeutic relationships and yet evidence is scarce regarding 'how to develop and sustain such relationships in a culture that increasingly focuses on throughput and rapid turnover' (Dewar and Nolan, 2013: 1247).

This is despite Lennart Fredriksson's publications on caring conversations in the late 1990s (Fredriksson, 1999). Fredriksson highlighted the need for intersubjectivity and how this facilitated comfort. He described nurses using their presence, touch and listening to provide compassionate care. Like Fredriksson, Dewar's conceptualisation of compassionate, relationship-centred care identifies the need for 'appreciative caring conversations'. For Dewar, these were based around two dimensions: 'Knowing who I am and what matters to me' and 'Understanding how I feel'. Parallels with the BOND framework (Baughan and Smith, 2013) are apparent in the model that Dewar developed, known as the 7Cs – this outlines the necessary factors to promote caring conversations:

- Being courageous
- Connecting emotionally
- Being curious
- Being collaborative
- Considering others' perspectives
- Compromising
- Being celebratory

David and Mary

On placement, I saw a 72-year-old gentleman called David accompanied by his wife and carer, Mary. David presented with a mixed-thickness scald to the fingers of his left hand. Mary explained to us that David had been diagnosed with dementia within the past year. David was unable to communicate effectively and Mary explained what had happened. David had gone upstairs to get ready for bed and a little while later she found him pulling at the damaged skin on his hand and concluded that he had turned on the hot tap and held his hand under the water.

We removed the dressing from David's hand and asked him to soak it in a bowl to soften any dead skin to be cut away. Whilst his hand was in the bowl, David started pulling the dead skin away. The nurse I was shadowing advised me to let David continue as David knew his own pain tolerance and it would be safer than if we were to use scissors.

Mary told me David had been in the Navy and travelled all over the world. During this time he had received medical training and Mary thought that was why David was removing the skin from his hand. I asked him to show me his best 'Navy' handshake, which distracted him.

The nurse asked David if he would like some painkillers and he did. I noticed that when taking them David drank the water very quickly so I offered him more. I then applied a dressing to David's hand and he assisted me by holding the dressings in place whilst I bandaged.

The nurse discussed with Mary how she was coping at home and whether they needed help. Mary explained that David had nursed her through cancer and she felt she should now care for him. We explained that it was important Mary considered her own health and occasional help would give her the rest to continue caring for David at home. The nurse advised Mary who to contact if she wanted to organise this.

Case study from Amy Scott

The nurses involved in David and Mary's care clearly developed a compassionate relationship with them within a short time. They were being **collaborative** in listening to and accepting Mary's explanation for why David was removing the damaged skin, as well as **courageous** in their confidence to let him do this, contrary to the usual protocols as this clinical judgement could be justified in the circumstances. The student was **curious** to learn about David, and Mary felt valued enough to disclose his experience in the Navy, enabling the student to **connect** emotionally and celebrate an important part of David's life by asking him to give her 'his best Navy handshake' (Figure 4.3). Finally, the nurse **considered** other perspectives by focusing on Mary's needs as well as David's and offering to organise some help at home, but reflecting on Mary's views, **compromised** by providing contact details for use should her situation change.

Model of culturally competent compassion: Papadopoulos (2014)

Papadopoulos (2014) acknowledges, as previous writers do, that compassion should be at the centre of contemporary healthcare. However, given the diversity of populations, she argues that the way compassionate care is demonstrated, perceived and received may

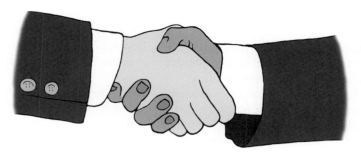

Figure 4.3   Navy handshake

differ due to the cultural background and experiences of the caregiver and recipient. Like Leininger (Leininger and MacFarland, 2006), Papadopoulos argues that cultural awareness and knowledge will inform our cultural sensitivity and empathy to ask appropriate questions to provide culturally competent care. She proposes a model for developing culturally compassionate healthcare professionals. This has four sequential stages arranged in a circle: *cultural awareness*, including universal understandings of compassion informed by philosophies and religion; this then informs *cultural knowledge* about similarities and differences in understanding compassion; together these encourage the practitioner to develop *cultural sensitivity* about giving and receiving compassion; and finally this enables *cultural competence* in the delivery of appropriate compassionate care. The model acknowledges that competence emerges over time and so each stage will be revisited again in different situations.

The need for person-centred compassionate care

Activity 4.4　Critical thinking

Why do you think person-centred compassionate care is important?

What evidence do you think might be available?

An outline answer is available at the end of the chapter.

Much of this chapter has highlighted the human imperative for person-centred compassionate care. Whilst it might be argued that this is an intrinsic trait of all human beings (Roach, 1987), or that caring skills need to be enhanced through education (Nightingale, 1859; Baughan and Smith, 2013), the culture of healthcare can inhibit practitioners from delivering this to patients (Francis, 2013). Person-centred compassionate care underpins healthcare practitioners' professional codes, but none the less it needs to become a central facet of our being to ensure this guides the way we practise.

However, compassionate care is not solely about humanising care; it also impacts on health outcomes. Street et al. (2009) explored the literature around the role of communication in healing. They suggest that effective clinician–patient communication improves health outcomes, directly and indirectly, through seven pathways: enabling access to care; increasing patient knowledge and encouraging shared understanding; enhancing the therapeutic alliance; enhancing patients' abilities to manage emotions; improving family and social support; enhancing patient empowerment and agency; and, lastly, facilitating higher-quality decisions. It would seem, therefore, that therapeutic relationships and effective communication are not simply optional extras but have physical and psychological benefits.

In the last few years, there has been extensive research interest in the effect of person-centred compassionate care. It has been identified that psychosocial well-being can be improved by effective communication where patients experience hope and feel known, validated, worthy, reassured and comforted (Thorne et al., 2005; Hack et al., 2005). Person-centred care improves quality of life and increases the ability to perform **activities of daily living** (Teitelman et al., 2010; Dudas et al., 2012; Sjogren et al., 2013) and experience increased well-being (Sloane et al., 2004; Bone et al., 2010; McKeown et al., 2010; Teitelman et al., 2010) and lowered agitation (Moniz Cook et al., 2003; Sloane et al., 2004; Chenoweth et al., 2009; Teitelman et al., 2010).

Chapter summary

This chapter explored the nature of compassionate care and its relationship with the culture of care, including the attitudes and approach of caregivers. It has been argued that, whilst the general public expect care to be compassionate, reports of contemporary practice have found that at times the focus on the person as the centre of care becomes secondary at the expense of fulfilling technical needs and organisational targets. This is despite some excellent models of care dating back to Victorian times, as we have seen, as well as more recent frameworks for compassionate care. Fortunately, the pendulum has swung back towards person-centred compassionate care and this is acknowledged not only by theorists but also significantly by policy-makers, as evidenced by the NHS nursing and midwifery strategy (the 6Cs) as well as the NHS Constitution. The psychological understanding of person-centred approaches will be explored further in the next chapter.

Further study

The website of *Frameworks 4 Change* offers some free resources to support self-compassion and a link to a talk on 'closing the compassion gap' by Andy Bradley, their founder. See: www.frameworks4change.co.uk/

To gain information and updates on compassionate care in the NHS, this website has links to policies and facilities to subscribe for updates: www.gov.uk/government/policies/compassionate-care-in-the-nhs/

Activity outline answers

Activity 4.1   Critical thinking

Think of a time when you were offered compassionate care or offered compassionate care to someone else. Make a few notes on what this looked and felt like.
It perhaps involved gentle touch, soft speech, kind words, taking time.
It perhaps felt good, peaceful, comfortable, okay, accepted, respected, acknowledged.

Activity 4.3   Creative thinking

Considering your notes from Activity 4.1, how would you define compassion?
Compassion involves facilitating both the carer and the person being cared for to feel respected, comfortable and accepted by the sharing of time, touch and supportive communication.

Activity 4.4 Critical thinking

Why do you think person-centred compassionate care is important?
What evidence do you think might be available?

You might suggest it is important to make the person feel comfortable and more accepting of care. Person-centred compassionate care underpins healthcare practitioners' professional codes but also impacts on health outcomes.

There is a wealth of research evidence which identifies the importance and need for this type of care. It has been identified that psychosocial well-being can be improved by effective communication where patients experience hope and feel known, validated, worthy, reassured and comforted (Thorne et al., 2005; Hack et al., 2005). Person-centred care improves quality of life and increases the ability to perform activities of daily living (Teitelman et al., 2010; Dudas et al., 2012; Sjogren et al., 2013); increased well-being (Sloane et al., 2004; Bone et al., 2010; McKeown et al., 2010; Teitelman et al., 2010); and experience lowered agitation (Moniz Cook et al., 2003; Sloane et al., 2004; Chenoweth et al., 2009; Teitelman et al., 2010).

References

Alderwick, H., Robertson, R., Appleby, J., Dunn, P. and Maguire, D. (2015) *Better Value in the NHS: The Role of Changes in Clinical Practice*. Available at: www.kingsfund.org.uk/sites/files/kf/field/field_publication_file/better-value-nhs-Kings-Fund-July2015.pdf (accessed 13 August 2015).

Barry, A.-M. and Yuill, C. (2008) *Understanding the Sociology of Health: An Introduction*. London: Sage.

Baughan, J. and Smith, A. (2013) *Compassion, Caring and Communication: Skills for Nursing Practice*, 2nd edn. London: Routledge.

Bolton, S.C. (2000) 'Who cares? Offering emotion work as a "gift" in the nursing labour process', *Journal of Advanced Nursing*, 32 (3): 580–6.

Bone, C., Cheung, G. and Wade, B. (2010) 'Evaluating person-centred care and dementia mapping in a psychogeriatric hospital in New Zealand', *New Zealand Journal of Occupational Therapy*, 57 (1): 35–40.

Brazier, C. (2003) *Buddhism on the Couch: From Analysis to Awakening, Using Buddhist Psychology*. Berkeley, CA: Ulysses Press – Seastone.

Chenoweth, L., King, M.T., Jeon, Y.-H., Brodaty, H., Stein-Parbury, J., Norman, R., Haas, M. and Luscombe, G. (2009) 'Caring for Aged Dementia Care Resident Study (CADRES) of person-centred care, dementia-care mapping, and usual care in dementia: A cluster-randomised trial', *The Lancet Neurology*, 8 (4): 317–25.

Department of Health (DH) (2008) *High Quality Care for All (Darzi Report)*. London: DH.

DH (2010) *Equity and Excellence: Liberating the NHS*. London: DH.

DH (2012) *Compassion in Practice*. Available at: www.england.nhs.uk/wp-content/uploads/2012/12/compassion-in-practice.pdf (accessed 12 August 2015).

DH (2013) *Patients First and Foremost: The Initial Government Response to the Report of the Mid Staffordshire NHS Foundation Trust Public Inquiry*. Available at: www.gov.uk/government/uploads/system/uploads/attachment_data/file/170701/Patients_First_and_Foremost.pdf (accessed 12 August 2015).

DH (2015) *The NHS Constitution*. Available at: www.gov.uk/government/uploads/system/uploads/attachment_data/file/448466/NHS_Constitution_WEB.pdf (accessed 12 August 2015).

DH and NHS Commissioning Board (2012) *Compassion in Practice: Nursing, Midwifery and Care Staff – Our Vision and Strategy*. Available at: www.england.nhs.uk/wp-content/uploads/2012/12/compassion-in-practice.pdf (accessed 12 August 2015).

Dewar, B. and Nolan, M. (2013) 'Caring about caring: Developing a model to implement compassionate relationship-centred care in an older-people care setting', *International Journal of Nursing Studies*, 50 (9): 1247–58.

Draper, P. and McSherry, W. (2007) 'Culture, religion and spirituality', in R. Nemo, B. Aveyard and H. Heath (eds), *Older People and Mental Health Nursing: A Handbook of Care*. Oxford: Blackwell, pp. 115–23.

Dudas, K., Olsson, L., Wolf, A., Swedberg, K., Taft, C., Schaufelberger, M. and Ekman, I. (2012) 'Uncertainty in illness among patients with chronic heart failure is less in person-centred care than in usual care', *European Journal of Cardiovascular Nursing*, 12 (6): 521–8.

Equality Act (2010) *What is the Equality Act?* Available at: www.equalityhumanrights.com/legal-and-policy/legislation/equality-act-2010/what-equality-act (accessed 12 August 2015).

Eriksson, K. (2002) 'Caring Science in a new key', *Nursing Science Quarterly*, 15 (1): 61–5.

Flynn, M. (2012) *Winterbourne View Hospital: A Serious Case Review: Summary*. Available at: http://hosted.southglos.gov.uk/wv/summary.pdf (accessed 12 August 2015).

Francis, R. (2013) *Report of the Mid Staffordshire NHS Foundation Trust Public Inquiry: Executive Summary*. Available at: www.gov.uk/government/uploads/system/uploads/attachment_data/file/279124/0947.pdf (accessed 12 August 2015).

Fredriksson, L. (1999) 'Modes of relating in a caring conversation: A research synthesis on presence, touch and listening', *Journal of Advanced Nursing*, 30 (5): 1167–76.

Freshwater, D. and Stickley, T. (2004) 'The heart of the art: Emotional intelligence in nurse education', *Nursing Inquiry*, 11 (2): 91–8.

Galvin, K. and Todres, L. (2013) *Caring and Well-Being: A Lifeworld Approach*. London: Routledge.

General Medical Council (GMC) (2013) *Good Medical Practice Guidance*. Available at: www.gmc-uk.org/guidance/good_medical_practice/duties_of_a_doctor.asp (accessed 12 August 2015).

GMC and Nursing and Midwifery Council (NMC) (2015) *Professional Duty of Candour*. Available at: www.nmc.org.uk/globalassets/sitedocuments/nmc-publications/openness-and-honesty-when-things-go-wrong–the-professional-duty-of-candour.pdf (accessed 12 August 2015).

Gilbert, P. (2009) 'Introducing compassion-focused therapy', *Advances in Psychiatric Treatment*, 15: 199–208.

Goetz, J.L., Keltner, D. and Simon-Thomas, E. (2010) 'Compassion: An evolutionary analysis and empirical review', *Psychological Review*, 136: 351–74.

Hack, T., Degner, L. and Parker, P. (2005) 'The communication goals and needs of cancer patients: A review', *Psychology*, 14: 831–45.

Hall, J. (2001) *Midwifery, Mind and Spirit: Emerging Issues of Care*. Oxford: Elsevier, Books for Midwives.

Health and Care Professions Council (HCPC) (2008) *Standards of Conduct, Performance and Ethics*. Available at: www.hpc-uk.org/aboutregistration/standards/standardsofconductperformanceandethics/ (accessed 12 August 2015).

John, V. and Parsons, E. (2006) 'Shadow work in midwifery: Unseen and unrecognised emotional labour', *British Journal of Midwifery*, 14 (5): 266–71.

Kendrick, K. and Robinson, S. (2002) '"Tender loving care" as a relational ethic in nursing practice', *Nursing Ethics*, 9 (3): 291–300.

Kirkup, B. (2015) *The Report of the Morecombe Bay Investigation*. Available at: www.bmj.com/content/346/bmj.f4017.full (accessed 12 August 2015).

Kitwood, T. (1997) *Dementia Reconsidered: The Person Comes First*. Maidenhead: Open University.

Lakeman, R., Cook, J. and McGowan, P. (2007) 'Service users, authority, power and protest: A call for renewed activism', *Mental Health Practice*, 11 (4): 12–16.

Leininger, M. (1991) *Cultural Care Diversity and Universality: A Worldwide Nursing Theory*. Sudbury, MA: Jones and Bartlett Publishers.

Leininger, M. and McFarland, M. (2006) *Cultural Care Diversity and Universality: A Worldwide Nursing Theory*, 2nd edn. Sudbury, MA: Jones and Bartlett Publishers.

MacBeth, A. and Gumley, A. (2012) 'Exploring compassion: A meta-analysis of the association between self-compassion and psychopathology', *Clinical Psychology Review*, 32: 545–52.

McKeown, J., Clarke, A., Ingleton, C., Ryan, T. and Repper, J. (2010) 'The use of life story work with people with dementia to enhance person-centered care', *International Journal of Older People Nursing*, 5 (2): 148–58.

MENCAP (2007) *Death by Indifference*. Available at: www.mencap.org.uk/sites/default/files/documents/2008-03/DBIreport.pdf (accesssed 12 August 2015).

MENCAP (2013) *Mencap Statement Regarding the Department of Health's Response to the Confidential Inquiry into Premature Deaths of People with a Learning Disability*. Available at: /www.mencap.org.uk/news/article/mencap-statement-regarding-department-health-s-response-confidential-inquiry-premature-deaths (accessed 12 August 2015).

Moniz-Cook, E., Stokes, G. and Agar, S. (2003) 'Difficult behaviour and dementia in nursing homes: five cases of psychosocial interventions', *Clinical psychology & psychotherapy*. 10 (3): 197-208

Morrison, P. (1992) *Professional Caring in Practice: A Psychological Analysis*. Aldershot: Avebury, Ashgate.

Napoles, A.M., Chadiha, L., Eversley, R. and Moreno-John, G. (2010) 'Developing culturally sensitive dementia caregiver interventions: Are we there yet?' *American Journal of Alzheimer's Disease and Other Dementias*, 25 (5): 389–406.

Nightingale, F. (1859) *Notes on Nursing: What it is and What it is Not*. London: Harrison.

Nursing and Midwifery Council (NMC) (2004) *Codes of Conduct for Nurses and Midwives*. London: NMC.

NMC (2009) *Guidance on Professional Conduct for Nursing and Midwifery Students*. Available at: www.health.herts.ac.uk/immunology/MentorshipUpdate/NMC Professional standarrds for student nurses and midwives.pdf (accessed January 2016).

NMC (2015) *The Code*. Available at: www.nmc.org.uk/globalassets/sitedocuments/nmc-publications/revised-new-nmc-code.pdf (accessed 12 August 2015).

Papadopoulos, I. (2014) *What is Culturally Competent Compassion?* Available at: http://cultureandcompassion.com/what-is-culturally-competent-compassion-2/ (accessed 6 August 2015).

Parliamentary and Health Service Ombudsman (2011) *Care and Compassion?* Available at: www.ombudsman.org.uk/__data/assets/pdf_file/0016/7216/Care-and-Compassion-PHSO-0114web.pdf (accessed 12 August 2015).

Roach, S. (1987) *The Human Act of Caring: A Blueprint for the Health Professions*. Ottawa: Canadian Healthcare Association Press.

Sjogren, K., Lindkvist, M., Sandman, P., Zingmark, K. and Edvardsson, D. (2013) 'Person-centredness and its association with resident well-being in dementia care units', *Journal of Advanced Nursing*, 69 (10): 2196–206.

Sloane, P.D., Hoeffer, B., Mitchell, C.M., Mckenzie, D.A., Barrick, A.L., Rader, J., Stewart, B.J., Talerico, K.A., Rasin, J.H., Zink, R.C. and Koch, G.G. (2004) 'Effect of person-centered showering and the towel bath on bathing-associated aggression, agitation, and discomfort in nursing home residents with dementia: A randomized, controlled trial', *Journal of the American Geriatrics Society*, 52 (11): 1795–804.

Social Care Institute for Excellence (SCIE) (2015) *Involving Service Users and Carers in Social Work Education*. Available at: www.scie.org.uk/publications/guides/guide04/gs/10-3.asp (accessed 12 August 2015).

Stickley, T. and Spandler, H. (2014) 'Compassion and mental health nursing', in T. Stickley and N. Wright (eds), *Theories for Mental Health Nursing: A Guide for Practice*. London: Sage, pp. 134–46.

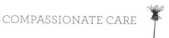

Street, R., Makoul, G., Neeraj, A. and Epstein, R. (2009) 'How does communication heal? Pathways linking clinician–patient communication to health outcomes', *Patient Education and Counseling*, 74: 295–301.

Teitelman, J., Raber, C. and Watts, J. (2010) 'The power of the social environment in motivating persons with dementia to engage in occupation: Qualitative findings', *Physical and Occupational Therapy Geriatrics*, 28 (4): 321–33.

Thorne, S., Armstrong, E., McPherson, G., Harris, S. and Hislop, T. (2005) '"Being known": Patients' perspectives of the dynamics of human connection in cancer care', *Psycho-Oncology*, 14: 887–98.

Thurgood, M. (2009) 'Engaging clients in their care and treatment', in I. Norman and I. Ryrie (eds), *The Art and Science of Mental Health Nursing: A Textbook of Principles and Practice*, 2nd edn. Maidenhead: Open University Press, McGraw-Hill Education, pp. 621–37.

Watson, J. (2007) *Human Science and Human Care: A Theory of Nursing*. Sudbury, MA: Jones and Bartlett Publishers.

Watson, J. (2010) *Caring Science Institute*. Available at: www.watsoncaringscience.org/ (accessed August 2015).

5 Person-Centred Approaches

Sue Barker

Breathe deep
Fly high
Seek peace

Learning objectives

This chapter's learning objectives are to:

- Identify the main philosophical influences in psychology
- Discuss what it is to be person-centred
- Explore the significance of person-centred approaches in contemporary society

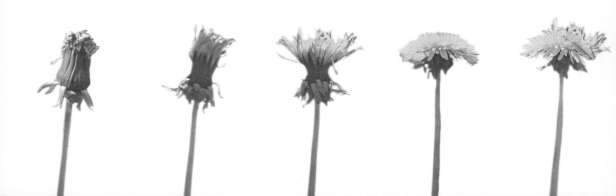

Introduction

In this book so far, we have explored what psychology is, along with its major theoretical frameworks. We have also examined the concept of compassionate care through the current culture of care and its scientific underpinning. This chapter will question the thinking which has led to the contemporary desire for compassionate care and how developing understanding in this area offers psychological support for compassionate care. This starts with an exploration of the philosophical underpinning of psychology.

It would therefore appear pertinent to define philosophy. A brief dictionary definition of philosophy is the 'love of wisdom', from the Greek word *philosophia* which can be divided up as *philo* ('love') and 'sophy' (knowledge or wisdom). For people with a more scientific inclination, philosophy is the love of knowledge, whereas for myself I prefer the phrase 'love of wisdom' which for me is a broader term. Having a doctorate in philosophy (PhD), my role is to teach or facilitate (*doctorate* is Latin for 'to teach') a love of wisdom or learning – a definition which I enjoy sharing with students.

Activity 5.1   Reflection

Sit somewhere comfortable and let your body relax. Work through your muscles, ensuring any tension is released. Listen to the sounds around you: you will maybe hear sounds from outside, perhaps traffic or birdsong, or you may hear sounds from inside the room such as a ticking clock or your own heartbeat. Listen to your breathing and just for a few moments experience your embodied self. Try to put on one side your previous knowledge and attitudes as you read through this chapter.

As this is a reflection, there is no outline answer at the end of the chapter.

Philosophical beginnings

Definitions of psychology have changed over time, despite psychology as a science being fairly young. Psychology is generally considered to have its genesis in the opening of Wilhelm Wundt's psychological laboratory in 1879 but others acknowledge Gustav Fechner's publication of the *Elemente der Psychophysik* in 1860 as the beginning of scientific psychology (Robinson, 2010).

The **etymology** of the word 'psychology' can easily be determined through contemporary dictionaries as deriving from the Greek language: *psyche* ('mind' or 'spirit') and *logos* ('study' or 'knowledge'). Therefore, literally, the word 'psychology' can be defined as the study of the mind/spirit or knowledge of the mind/spirit. Whilst this sounds simple, understandings of mind and spirit are culturally influenced and differ over time as with any cultural **concept**.

'Mind' can be explained through mental processes such as problem-solving, object perception and communication. It can, though, also be considered to be an object or structure: the repository of information and knowledge such as memory. For others still, the mind is recognised as a motivating force prompting behaviour, emotions and thoughts. How the mind is understood has been and will continue to be considered as we progress through this book, as each psychological perspective offers a different explanation.

The mind has been accepted as something that can be explored, examined and explained scientifically, which is probably why psychologists have focused on this term rather than the other word that can be used for psyche: spirit. In the late nineteenth and the twentieth centuries, when scientific psychologists were establishing their field of practice and developing their grand theories, there was little attention given to study of the spirit in healthcare in Western societies. This may be due to spirit being linked to 'soul', a non-physical element of the person that many believe will survive after the body dies, and also spirituality being linked to theology. Theology, 'the study of God', is not usually considered to be a science, and the early psychologists were keen to be recognised as and gain the status of scientists.

Contemporary views of the spirit are still that it is a non-physical concept, with Verity and Lee (2011) suggesting that the spirit is the 'spark of life' in people. Spirituality has been defined as: 'That which lies at the core of each person's being, an essential dimension which brings meaning to life' (MacKinlay, 2001: 52). MacKinlay (2011) identifies, in her model of spirituality adapted for those with dementia, that transcending loss and finding hope and intimacy with god or in relationship with others are significant features which interact with a sense of meaning for the person. It is therefore easy to see why scientific psychological researchers have more frequently used the word 'mind' when explaining what they do.

For thousands of years, prior to the opening of Wundt's laboratory, the mind had been explored by philosophers. The earliest philosopher to directly influence psychology was probably Aristotle (384–322 BCE) who argued that everything had four causes: material (what it is made of); formal (what it is); efficient (what makes it); and final (its purpose). He offered us terms such as **'substance'**, **'essence'** and **'energy'**, and processes such as 'categorisation' to talk about and organise the science of psychology. The divination of philosophical thought over the years can also be seen to influence the development of psychology. The most prominent are the philosophies of rationalism (particularly Descartes' **dualism**) and **empiricism** (particularly Locke's *tabula rasa*, Hume's positivism and Berkeley's **idealism**). The early schools of psychology from which the contemporary psychological perspectives are based can be seen as a development of philosophical thought and understanding of the person.

The three major early underpinning philosophies were:

- *Animism*: Everything in the world has purpose; everything is influenced by its mind or spirit, including the sun, the trees and the sea
- *Rationalism*: All knowledge comes from the mind. René Descartes (1596–1650) stated that mind and matter (body) were separate entities but only humans possessed a mind. This theory was called 'dualism'
- *Empiricism*: Knowledge or understanding can only be gained through observation and experience. John Locke (1632–1704) identified the infant as being a blank slate (*tabula rasa*), stating it had no experience and therefore did not know anything. George Berkeley (1685–1753) went on to state that all knowledge comes from the senses, which was labelled 'idealism'. David Hume (1711–76) further developed empirical thought by adopting a 'positivist' philosophy, only accepting evidence that was observable and measurable to understand people – see the theory box on 'Philosophical underpinning of psychology'.

Philosophical underpinning of psychology

Ancient Greek philosophers
The ancient Greek philosophers offered ideas related to faith, ethics and what it means to be a person. The main people were:

> Pythagoras (*c.* 580–500 BCE), Socrates (469–399 BCE), Plato (*c.* 429–*c.* 347 BCE) and Aristotle (384–322 BCE)

Hellenistic and Roman periods
This period produced a number of schools that developed on from the ancient Greeks but also saw the development of:

> Epicureanism through Epicurus (341–270 BCE), which was to disappear; and eclecticism by Cicero (106–43 BCE), which can still be seen to be relevant today

Mediaeval period
This era mostly accepted the philosophy of the ancient Greeks. It was a time of focusing on faith, reason, existence and knowledge but was influenced by Christian and Arabic theology among others – such as:

> *Christian*: St Francis of Assisi (*c.* 1182–1226) and Aquinas (*c.* 1221–74); *Islamic*: Al-Razi (*c.* 865–925); *Judaism*: Maimonides (*c.* 1135–1204); and *humanist*: Giovanni Pico della Mirandola (1463–94)

Early modern period
The period from the Renaissance (1400s–1700) to the time of Enlightenment (1700s) saw a resurgence of interest in the ancient Greek philosophers, with a major philosophical force at this time being the humanists such as Erasmus (1466–1536) and Thomas More (1478–1535). But this was a time of exploring the nature of knowledge and reason, with the two main groups divided into empiricists and rationalists:

> *Empiricists*: Francis Bacon (1561–1626), John Locke (1632–1704), David Hume (1711–76) and George Berkeley (1685–1753)

> *Rationalists*: René Descartes (1596–1650), Baruch de Spinoza (1632–77) and Nicolas Malebranche (1638–1715)

Modern period
After the time of the Enlightenment, the ancient Greek philosophers and their successors have led to numerous categories of philosophical exploration in modern times.

Analytical empiricists basically follow empirical philosophy but diverge from the early empiricists by offering a logical technique to achieve definitive answers. They include:

(Continued)

(Continued)

Bertrand Russell (1872–1970), G.E. Moore (1873–1958) and Karl Popper (1902–94)

Logical positivists/empiricists can be seen as analytical empiricists but they stressed that everything deduced should be verifiable through observation; they included:

Hans Reichenbach (1891–1953) and Kurt Grelling (1886–1942)

Idealists reject empirical science, suggest that reality cannot be known, all of our experience is in our mind. Idealists included:

Immanuel Kant (1724–1804) and Friedrich Wilhelm Joseph Schelling (1775–1854)

Existentialists suggest that any search for knowledge should begin within the person: we need to understand individual experiences. These included:

Søren Kierkegaard (1813–55), Friedrich Nietzsche (1844–1900), Martin Buber (1878–1965) and Jean-Paul Sartre (1905–80)

Phenomenologists identify that there are essential realities but people are always focused on the object and so are unable to recognise the essence of the phenomenon:

Franz Brentano (1838–1917), Edmund Husserl (1859–1938), Martin Heidegger (1889–1976) and Maurice Merleau-Ponty (1908–61)

Pragmatists recognise the need for empirical study but the need also to see how that relates to real-world experience and relationships:

William James (1842–1910) and John Dewy (1859–1952)

The first school of scientific psychology was called **structuralism. School** here means a collection of people who think about things in a similar way, not an educational establishment. The school of structuralism was established through the work of Wilhelm Wundt and is called 'structuralism' because it focuses on the structure of the mind. Wundt's experimental work used **introspection** to discover the essential elements of the mind. Wundt and his colleagues did this to develop their understanding of these elements in the same way other sciences had identified essential elements such as the periodic table in chemistry. However, the use of introspection to understand the mind could be labelled a rationalist approach, which was unacceptable to those who understood the world through empiricism, particularly the positivists. This school was therefore problematic philosophically.

The next school of psychology to be created was called **functionalism**. This was led by the empiricists and was influenced by the writings of the evolutionary scientist Charles Darwin (1809–82). They were interested in the function of the mind, not internal individual thoughts. They sought to find out how the mind operated (functioned), not how it was arranged (structure). Structuralism, as a school, no longer exists in any contemporary psychological perspective unless we accept the biopsychological under-standing of localisation of the brain as the structure of the mind. Functionalism can, though, clearly be seen in the psychological perspectives of behaviourism and cognitive psychology. This underlying empirical approach to psychology guides scientists to rec-ognise that all people biologically function the same and that there is no difference between mind and body – all people have evolved in reaction to environmental influences.

Scientific approach

It is perhaps important that we consider what the scientific approach is at this point. The scientific approach, derived from empiricism, has a method for developing under-standing and a format for presenting findings.

1. Identify the problem – formulate hypothesis
2. Design the experiment – to test the hypothesis by managing the variables
3. Conduct the experiment – observations are recorded
4. Evaluate the hypothesis through analysis of the data
5. Communicate the results

The format for presenting findings using the scientific approach is:

1. Title
2. Abstract
3. Introduction
4. Method
5. Results
6. Discussion
7. References
8. Appendices

As will become apparent later in this chapter, this structured scientific approach is not useful for all psychological perspectives, particularly stages 2 and 3, but it is estab-lished as the primary philosophy for developing contemporary knowledge globally. The hierarchy of research findings values these empirical studies most highly.

Other philosophical and biological theories were developing during the nineteenth and twentieth centuries that were to influence the development of contemporary psychological perspectives. Freud was a student of Franz Brentano (1838–1917), a philosopher at the same time as Edmund Husserl (1859–1938), considered to be the founding father of philosophical phenomenology and a radical idealist (see the the-ory box on 'Philosophical underpinning of psychology'). Both Freud and Husserl rejected dualism and accepted the mind as having a psychic energy outside of the material body. This philosophical approach, along with physiology and medicine, particularly psychiatry, influenced Freud's psychodynamic/psychoanalytic theory, which has become the psychodynamic perspective (one of the modern schools of psychology; see Chapter 1). Phenomenological and existential philosophy alongside psychodynamic, behavioural and cognitive psychological approaches all impacted on the development of the later humanist perspective in psychology (another school of modern psychology; see Chapter 1).

Philosophical thought as well as other developing theories from areas such as biology, anthropology and sociology continue to be used by psychologists to support their developing understanding through their own research. Indeed, there are large overlaps in the interests of psychologists, and other scientists and some psychologists have incorporated other disciplines to define their theoretical standpoint, such as social psychologists and biopyschologists.

Given the proliferation of schools or approaches within psychology, different texts will offer a different set of perspectives but those generally accepted are behaviourist, cognitivist, humanist, psychodynamic and biologist. As psychology has developed into a modern science, the way in which it defines itself has also changed.

Historical definitions of psychology

Early definitions of psychology all derive from those developing a scientific understanding of the mind or soul, hence the establishment of the word 'psychology'. This, of course, leads to definitions derived from a scientific philosophical approach; they are concerned with defining and describing what they are doing and why. This would exclude definitions from rationalists, phenomenologists and existentialists as they were not recognised as following the scientific method.

William James (1842–1910), a pragmatist that accepted the need for empirical understanding like Hume, was considered an important proponent of the development of functionalism. In 1890, he offered one of the earliest definitions of psychology: 'the science of mental life both of its phenomena and of their conditions ... The phenomena are such things as we call feelings, desires, cognition, reasoning, decision and the like' (James, 1890: 1). Interestingly, James refers to the term 'soul' as well as 'mind' in his explanation of what psychology is, demonstrating his pragmatism.

John B. Watson (1878–1958) was philosophically based in empiricism and positivism but he was significantly influenced by the functionalist approach of James. In 1919, Watson (Gross, 2005: 4) offered a definition of psychology as: 'that division of Natural Science which takes human behaviour – the doings and sayings, both learned and unlearned – as the subject matter'. Watson can be seen as the founder of the school of behaviourism within psychology. He developed his theories and research in the same era as Thorndike (1874–1949), an animal behaviourist, and Pavlov (1849–1936), a physiologist, who both provided behavioural psychologists with theories supported by scientific empirical evidence.

During the same period of the twentieth century, Freud (1856–1939) was developing his understanding of the mind, initially through neurology but later through philosophy and psychiatry. As Freud's exploration of the mind involved introspection and observations of patients, it did not 'fit' the scientific philosophy of the era and at this time his work was not part of the psychological establishment. Therefore, no recorded definition of psychology is available from him but he did provide us with a large volume of written descriptions of the mind. Freud saw the mind as a dynamic structure and force; it has a biological basis but is influenced by experiences, particularly early life relationships (see Chapters 1 and 2).

In the mid-twentieth century, humanistic psychology was developing as a reaction against psychodynamic thought and behaviourism. The humanists, as with the psychodynamic psychologists, did not accept a purely scientific approach to understanding the mind so we do not have a precise definition of psychology from them, but they do give us an understanding of the mind that builds on phenomenological and existential philosophy along with psychodynamic and behavioural psychology. They see the mind or human nature as being positive and creative with the power and potential for individual growth.

At the beginning of the twenty-first century, there continues to be debate between those who seek to understand the mind, with Carlson et al. (2004: 4) defining psychology as: 'the science of behaviour ... the word "psychology" literally means – the science of the mind'. This is supported by other commentators such as Gerrig et al. (2012: 4), who state that psychology can be defined as 'the scientific study of the behaviour of individuals and their mental processes'. This fits well with the definition given by the British Psychological Society (2015), the professional body for psychologists in Britain: 'Psychology is the scientific study of people, the mind and behaviour.'

The American Psychological Society (2015) has attempted to offer a more inclusive definition of psychology whilst accepting the definitions provided above. They state on their website that:

Psychology is the study of the mind and behavior. The discipline embraces all aspects of the human experience – from the functions of the brain to the actions of nations, from child development to care for the aged. In every conceivable setting from scientific research centers to mental healthcare services, 'the understanding of behavior' is the enterprise of psychologists.

We can still see, though, that the psychological establishment remains embedded within empirical scientific philosophy.

All theorists and researchers will have their personal worldview; in my opinion, these worldviews will lead them to interpret and explain concepts such as the mind and soul in different ways. The ongoing use of the scientific philosophical approach indicates contemporary bias in understanding the mind. These worldviews are called 'ideologies' by sociologists, but other psychologists who accept a worldview that is more phenomenological and humanistic but still empirical in its broadest sense may find the following definition of psychology useful:

Psychology seeks to understand why people behave, think and feel the way they do individually and in groups in all areas of life including health. Psychologists not only seek to predict behaviour but also to change behaviours to enhance well-being and quality of life. (Barker, 2007: 3)

Activity 5.2   Reflection

Take a few minutes to think about what you have read. Is your understanding of psychology the same as when you started this chapter or has it changed?

How would you define psychology?

As this is a reflection, there is no outline answer at the end of the chapter.

Given the definitions provided here, we can see that there is a well-established group of psychologists who identify psychology as the science of the mind. There are, though, those who seek a more encompassing understanding which incorporates other philosophical approaches such as existentialism. To understand the phenomenon of compassion (see Chapter 4) as well as the behaviour of compassionate care, the writings of Amedeo Giorgi can be seen to be useful, especially his development of phenomenological psychology, along with the work of philosophical psychologists Eugene Gendlin and Les Todres; their work will be explored in more detail later in this chapter.

Summary

Health and social care practitioners can and do use psychological research and theories to enhance their practice, and most caring practices have a foundation in philosophy, psychology, sociology or biology. Although most care practitioners have now developed their own unique bodies of knowledge, other approaches can still enhance their understanding and practice.

Person-centred

There is no single precise definition of the term 'person-centred care'. This is partly due to it still being an emerging and evolving concept. The Health Foundation (2014) has, though, identified a framework that comprises four principles of person-centred care:

1. Affording people dignity, compassion and respect
2. Offering coordinated care, support or treatment
3. Offering personalised care, support or treatment
4. Supporting people to recognise and develop their own strengths and abilities to enable them to live an independent and fulfilling life

Similarly, the Royal College of Nursing (2015) outlines that the key concepts that combine to make person-centred care are:

- Respect and holism
- Power and empowerment
- Choice and autonomy
- Empathy and compassion

Likewise, the Health Care Professions Council (2014) state that:

When asked what a good experience of care looked like, participants described professionals who were 'person centred' and passionate about their work. Technical competence in the absence of a genuinely personalised approach was not enough.

The British Psychological Society (2013) also recognised the importance of person-centre care and said that: 'Providing support and training to staff to recognise the difficulties faced by those with memory problems and to support them during hospital admissions is not difficult but does require a shift towards greater person-centred care.'

Morrissey and Callaghan (2011: 91) tell us that to be person-centred, we need to:

- Appreciate that each person is unique
- Believe that people are doing their best
- Respect the worthiness of each individual
- Behave genuinely and honestly
- Enable control to remain with the person
- Recognise that all people have needs and are motivated by them
- Realise that all behaviour is communicating something

It is important that a distinction is made between person-centred care and other types of care. Morse and her colleagues undertook many studies exploring how nurses responded to cues of suffering. They found that these could be divided into two categories: nurse-focused and patient-focused (Morse et al., 1992). These two categories could be subdivided into two more subcategories: taught and automatic.

Where nurses were focused on their role and the tasks they needed to undertake and had not received teaching on communication skills they exhibited behaviours including: guarding, dehumanising, withdrawing, distancing and labelling when confronted with suffering. When the nurse had received skills training, their behaviour was observed to be: rote or mechanical responses, false pity, false reassurance and offering closure statements such as 'don't worry'.

However, when the nurse was focusing on the person, they were person-centred; their automatic untaught behaviours were emotionally and culturally driven; and they unconsciously offered pity, sympathy, consolation, compassion, commiseration and reflexive reassurance. Furthermore, after person-centred communication skills education they were described as sharing something of themselves, sometimes confronting, sometimes using humour and giving informative reassurance (Morse et al., 1992).

Person

An exploration of personality theories can be found in Chapter 6 but it is important to reconsider the person or individual here. Uniqueness and individuality have an important philosophical position in Western cultures, as seen in the previous section, but as with other values and beliefs they have been adopted as our culture has developed. It is only in the last couple of hundred years that to view people as individuals has been the accepted norm in our culture.

 Agatha Wright

Case study

I was born during the Second World War; my father had been conscripted just after my mother got pregnant and was sent overseas. My first few years were spent in my maternal family home and I was mostly cared for by my grandmother and extended family, as every able-bodied person had to work and my mother had been sent to work in the aeroplane factory. There were no men in the family home except my grandfather and my cousin Wayne. I remember it as a happy time although I was told there was little money and food

(Continued)

(Continued)

was limited, and I do recall rationing books. I also recall how the family used to try to find additional ways of getting extra food. I remember one of my uncles being killed and how my grandmother would not talk about it. She stopped smiling after that; I wanted to make her happy but was unable to.

About a year after the war ended, I met my father for the first time at the age of five. He did not seem happy and grumbled that I was dirty – I had been out playing in the road with my cousin.

Life changed significantly on my father's return. My mother, father and I moved into a terraced house with two rooms upstairs and two rooms downstairs; unlike today's houses, it did not have a bathroom and the toilet was outside. My parents were to live there for the rest of their lives; after a while my brother was born. My father seemed stern but when he smiled; it was wonderful but this did not happen often. He would not talk about the war. Although I loved him he frightened me a bit. He also seemed to give my brother everything he wanted but was strict with me. I went to school but I was not a good scholar and looked forward to leaving. At 15, I got a job in a shop which I really enjoyed, and at 17 met my husband-to-be. He was handsome and strong and seemed very clever. My parents did not seem to like him very much; later I recognised why this might be. He has always been very controlling of me. Like my father, I was a bit frightened of my husband but when he smiled and touched me it was wonderful.

I quickly had two children after we were married, which made me very tired, and I had to visit my mother every week to help her with her shopping. This continued until she died when I reached 68 years of age. In her last few years, my mother had been quite demanding as my father died shortly after retiring. I also retired from my job as a hospital cleaner at 68 due to ill health. I now enjoy knitting, watching the television and seeing my grandchildren and great-grandchildren.

Activity 5.3   Critical thinking

Read the case study of Agatha Wright. How would you describe her personality? What do you think has influenced this?

There is an outline answer at the end of the chapter.

The concepts of 'person' and 'personhood' have been used and scrutinised within personality theories through a humanistic psychological lens. This way of understanding the person does not use inventories or behavioural checklists: it is about getting to know the person and how they understand themselves and give meaning to their lives. This is frequently seen as the person's spirituality which links mind and soul.

If we read the case study of Agatha, we can see what is important to her and what makes her distinct from others. Recognising oneself as different from others is how personhood is established. Agatha clearly demonstrated in her story that a key element of how she sees herself is in relationship with others. All of her narrative revolves around her family and their feelings and her feelings towards them. As the case study on Matthew Tracey shows, his story about himself and his life is quite different.

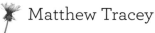 Matthew Tracey

I grew up in a happy family and I think this has been of benefit to me throughout my life. We were given lots of opportunities for education and plenty of support for whatever we were interested in. I do not think we had lots of money but it was used in an economic way. We moved several times when I was a child but this did not concern me; in fact, I think it prepared me well for adult life where I have had to move houses to access job opportunities.

At school I did well and it was expected I would attend university, which I did. I was a little nonconformist in that my highest grades at school had been in the sciences; my parents I think hoped I would become an engineer. I chose to study mathematics. I left with an average degree but given I had spent a fair amount of time in the rugby club this was no surprise.

I got a job after my first degree with an established accountancy firm and I have been fortunate as they provided good career development opportunities. I became chartered after three years and gained a Master's a few years later. I established my own firm a few years ago, which I have seen grow. I mostly now act as an advisor and use my golfing hobby as a networking opportunity.

I have been married for 30 years and have two children. I am very proud of their achievements; they are independent and successful young people.

Activity 5.4   Critical thinking

After you have read Matthew's story, identify the significant factors that you will need to take into consideration when caring for him.

There is an outline answer at the end of the chapter.

Matthew's story is quite different and we can see that he has highlighted different aspects of himself that he wants others to know. He identified personal characteristics such as independence and intelligence; he also highlights his achievements – professional, academic and personal (houses, children and business).

If care practitioners listen to people's stories, they can identify how the person sees themselves, what is important and gives their lives meaning, and what might motivate them towards recovery or a sense of well-being.

Within the humanistic psychological view developed by Rogers (see Chapter 1), self-concept is central to the person's understanding of themselves which is crucial for personal growth and fulfilment of potential. A person's self-concept is made up of **self-worth** or esteem, **self-image** and **ideal self**. The closer the self-image and ideal self are, the higher the self-worth or esteem is. This allows the self-concept to be congruent: the person being genuine and honest with themselves and others. This is achieved through the child's needs for positive regard from those close to them, leading to self-worth or esteem.

Self-concept is based on the individual's **phenomenological field**, of which we had a small snapshot with Agatha and Matthew. This is their subjective experience of the world, which is always changing. The person's world (phenomenological field) is their perception of their experiences. This differs from their **perceptual field,** in that the phenomenological field incorporates the perceptual field but also includes other types of awareness and knowing, for example spiritual awareness and aesthetic knowing. Their perceptual field provides the person with a sense of reality; it is their personal 'reality'. This reality is the only reality available to the person (see Chapters 1 and 6).

Activity 5.5   Critical thinking

In mental healthcare, some people are described as 'not being in touch with reality', as they are diagnosed with an illness that means they are experiencing delusions. Look at the list below and decide which of these thoughts might be delusional:

I have an angel that looks after me

I have conversations with God

I am more intelligent than you

I have a sixth sense: I know when something bad is going to happen

I am famous

I am a disgusting person

An outline answer is given at the end of the chapter.

The person's emotions, values and beliefs are significant factors in their perception of their phenomenological field. They may experience a greater sense of themselves when all their sensory and visceral experiences can be assimilated: their experiences are embodied. Rogers (1961: 189) writes that a person needs to 'open their spirit' to all of life's possibilities: the possibility of experiencing the rich tapestry of emotions and existential being.

Rogers (1961: 187–89) identified a fully functioning person as:

- Having an increasing openness to experience
- Increasingly developing existential living
- Increasing trust in their organism

A fully functioning person is always in a state of movement; they are always developing and changing. To be fully functioning and to have a good life Rogers (1961: 192–96) goes on to state that the process of the good life is to:

- Recognise our freedom of choice
- Be creative
- Trust in human nature
- Recognise the richness of life

The theory of Rogers, whilst based in phenomenology and existentialism, was – he believed – open to empirical research. This has been developed by others such as Kitwood in his person-centred care for people with dementia.

Personhood

Personhood can be seen to be the central concept in Kitwood's person-centred care; he defines it as 'a standing or status that is bestowed on one human being, by another, in the context of relationship and social being' (Kitwood, 1997: 8). Kitwood believes providing personhood facilitates the person being valued and treated with respect. The life world experiences for the person can be divided into three categories: personal characteristics, associated health state and **affiliation**.

Kitwood, in his model of person-centred care for people with dementia, identified five psychological needs of the person which occur in either a social malignant psychological environment or a positive person work environment. These psychological needs he organised into a flower (see Figure 3.1). He depicted the environment as two lists of 17 opposing behaviours – malignant social psychology was outlined in Chapter 3 (see Table 3.1). The attributes of positive person work can be seen in Table 5.1.

Table 5.1   Positive person work

Positive person work/carer behaviour	Example
Recognition	Welcoming the person by their name and introducing yourself by name
Negotiation	The person would like to go out to a coffee shop but you are waiting for a telephone call. You discuss with them if they can wait until you have received the call or whether you can answer your mobile phone whilst you are out together
Collaboration	It is one of the family's birthday, so you collaborate with the person on how and what cake to make or buy for them
Play	This could be something seated like bingo or more active like miniature golf, or it could be as simple as playing with words
Timalation	These can be a type of therapeutic touch, so an example could be massaging moisturiser onto a person's hand
Celebration	Recognising and identifying when someone has something to celebrate and providing the opportunity to do this
Relaxation	Giving time and space for relaxation, when a person does not feel under pressure to do anything or could be supported through relaxation
Validation	Recognising how a person feels and not being dismissive of it
Holding	Could be psychological such as sitting with a person whilst they are struggling with a thought or emotion, or it could be physical such as holding their hand
Facilitation	This is helping the person achieve what is important to them, e.g. attending a church service
Creation	Providing the opportunity for the person to be creative, whether mentally in conversation, artistically or making something practical like a cup of tea or cake
Giving	This is again providing the opportunity for the person to give something to someone else to feel that they have a purpose. It could be asking them to listen to a child read, or giving someone a message or advice

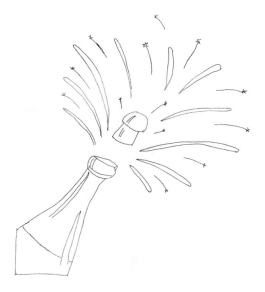

Figure 5.1   Celebration

Table 5.1 provides a list, with examples, of positive person work and whilst for most of them, such as relaxation, the impact on a sense of well-being may be obvious, for others this is less so. Play and celebration may appear less important. Whilst play can be motivating, both play and celebration can facilitate a feeling of pleasure; more significantly celebration can bring a sense of success leading to self-efficacy and self-esteem.

To be a person therefore would appear to be a sense of what gives yourself life meaning: to understand your own phenomenological field, to recognise the possibilities for your life and to make choices to grow towards these. Personhood appears to be something that is bestowed on another person (positive person work): it is where one person facilitates the other to be the person they have the possibility to become.

As care practitioners we therefore need to be congruent ourselves and to help others towards congruence. We can achieve this through the techniques identified by Kitwood in Table 5.1 and Rogers and Egan in Chapter 7. This is achievable and recommended in care environments through person-centred care.

Summary

Person-centred care is recommended by all governmental and professional bodies in the UK (DH, National Institute for Health and Care Excellence (NICE), SCIE, NMC, GMC, HCPC and BPS). Whilst it is a cultural phenomenon, it has been underpinned by philosophical thought and psychological theory. Frameworks for compassionate care, philosophical ideas and psychological theory continue to develop. Contemporary understandings of person-centred compassionate care that are supported by all of these are explored in the next section.

Contemporary psychological understanding of person-centred compassionate care

The development of person-centred compassionate care, despite the expectation of its provision within care services, is slowly progressing due to research funding bodies preferring to sponsor qualitative studies that produce quantifiable results. However, there have been some interesting developments based on the philosophical approaches of the phenomenologists and existentialists. Contemporary phenomenologists such as psychologist Les Todres and his colleague Kathleen Galvin, a nurse, have built on the foundations of Husserl, Heidegger, Merleau-Ponty, Gadama, Giorgi (psychologist) and Gendlin (psychologist).

Galvin and Todres identified, whilst engaging with philosophical thought and their health-related research, that something significant was missing in healthcare.

They identified this as a lack of attention to the 'things that make us feel more human' (Galvin and Todres, 2013). Adopting a life world approach based on phenomenological philosophy, psychology and healthcare, they developed the Humanising Values Framework (HVF) (see theory boxes 'Humanisation of care' and 'Forms of dehumanisation of care') which emphasises the values that should underpin authentic person-centred healthcare.

Humanising Values Framework (HVF)

Galvin and Todres proposed eight dimensions for humanising care. These were expressed as polemic values moving between the poles of dehumanising care to humanising care. Through their research, they have applied this approach to a number of clinical settings as well as professional education.

Humanisation of care (Todres et al., 2009)

- *Insiderness*: A person's subjectivity – their personal inside view of the world. Humanised care is care in which you acknowledge this and are respectful of the person's **perceptual world**
- *Agency*: This is where the person has the ability to make and be responsible for their own decisions/choices. To offer humanised care, you should facilitate the person's individuality, ensuring that they can make their own choices
- *Uniqueness*: The people we care for are more than the sum of their parts; they are different from others and therefore you should not expect everyone to behave the same or want the same things
- *Togetherness*: We exist in relationship with others; isolation can be a huge problem for the cared for as well as carers. To humanise your care you need to recognise that being with family and friends is important and consider how you can facilitate this through negotiation
- *Sense-making*: Our need and ability to find meaning and patterns in our world. For some this involves organised worship. To humanise your care, you need to consider how your sense of the world impacts on others and how you can help them make sense of what is happening to them
- *Personal journey*: This is a term that refers to our lifespan development – we develop, grow and change as we move along our life line. Our individual journeys are different and we have our own goals. As a care practitioner you should find out the goals that people you care for have, so that you can enhance their ability to achieve them
- *Sense of place*: Our sense of belonging, our experience of being at home. When you are caring for someone, it may be in their home where they feel they belong and are comfortable, but sometimes you need to organise the place they have to be (hospital, residential home, hospice) into somewhere they can experience this. This might include personal belongings, pets or people

(Continued)

(Continued)

- *Embodiment*: This refers to our experience of living: our perceptions, feelings and inter-actions. The experiences, perception, interactions and feelings of a person should not be denied or denigrated: they are what they say they are. As a care practitioner listen to the person's expression of these and try to address any needs that occur due to them

Forms of dehumanisation of care (Todres et al., 2009)

- *Objectification*: Could be where you ignore or deny the person's subjective experience – for example, they state that they are disturbed at night by people banging their front gate but you ignore this
- *Passivity*: Occurs by you making choices/decisions on behalf of the person and they then become passive by accepting your authority
- *Homogenisation*: This is where you expect all people to behave, think and feel the same and you therefore treat them the same
- *Isolation*: Could be where you restrict a person's social engagement opportunities – for example, restrictive visiting, excluded access to social groups or facilities
- *Loss of meaning*: Could occur intentionally or unintentionally when you ignore confu-sion or expressed loss of meaning, or make changes without explaining adequately
- *Loss of personal journey*: Can occur through a lack of recognition of the person's goals, hopes and expectations, as despite the lack of optimal health some may still be achieved. For example, the person with dementia would like to go out to a restaurant for a meal but you deny this due to their dementia
- *Dislocation*: This could occur if the person needs to move to a different care location such as a nursing home, or their condition deteriorates and the impact of this is not addressed
- *Reductionist body*: This could occur for the person if their expressions of pain or dis-comfort are dismissed instead of being investigated as it is assumed that all of their expressions are distorted due to the health problem

The framework guides care practitioners in their person-centred humanised care. This is achieved through some of the key philosophical concepts already identified, but they have offered further clarification of these and how they may be achieved. The terms they have used in their exploration are: 'insiderness', 'being with that' or 'embodied rela-tional understanding', 'empathic knowing', 'open-heartedness' and 'dwelling mobility'.

Insiderness

Insiderness is the understanding of the person's individual experiences or 'life world'. From its earliest inception person-centred approaches have all recognised that the starting point for understanding another person is to have a good understanding of ourselves: self-awareness. Rogers' stipulation for congruence requires that we are not only aware of our thoughts, feelings and experiences but also comfortable with ourselves: 'We are comfortable in our own skin'.

Todres et al. (2014) highlight three aspects to caring for insiderness, caring for the person and their life world, which are:

- 'Insiderness' always recedes from the view of the other person so that it can never be grasped absolutely
- 'Reaching towards' the 'insiderness' of another as a process and practice is often more important than 'knowing' the details of someone's 'insiderness'
- 'Caring for insiderness' calls for the complex use of self through 'reflective open-heartedness' and through life world knowledge as an interpretive touchstone

Insiderness at its simplest level could be identified as empathy but Gilbert, a scientific psychologist, as well as Todres, a phenomenological psychologist, recognises that there is more to the person and compassion than empathy. Insiderness is an awareness of and giving space to the person's phenomenological field – their whole life world experiences.

Being with that: embodied relational understanding

Carers need to make judgements or decisions when caring for others and 'embodied relational understanding' can facilitate them in working in a humanised person-centred way, which Todres has called 'being with that' (Todres, 2008). He used Hans-Georg Gadamer's, Maurice Merleau-Ponty's and Eugene Gendlin's writings to explain how 'being with that' or 'embodied relational understanding' could assist practitioners.

Gadamer indicated that we should be focused on the 'that' and not be disturbed by any of our internal preoccupations. He does not suggest this is to exclude one's sense of self, as we are all relational and cannot help responding to the other; he says that we have a 'bond' with the other person. Gendlin identifies that being embodied is essential for bonding in a similar way to Erikson's assertion that we need to develop our self-identify before we can engage in intimate relationships with others. Todres says that this bond resonates with the other person involving heart and empathy in judgements. This allows the practitioner to access and use all their embodied resources in the interaction, making the relationship feel open and alive.

Further to this, Gendlin (1962, 1992) guides us to recognise that 'sense-making' requires a knowing within our body; it is this that connects us to the world of experiences. Sense-making in this context is not only logical and factual, but also has a texture: 'the senses, the flesh, the histories, and multiple meanings' (Todres, 2007: 20) – this is a **felt sense** and more than words can say (Gendlin, 1962, 1992).

Therefore Todres leads us to understand that 'embodied relational understanding', knowing the other person through understanding our whole perceptual experiences and our bond with them, through a felt sense, will guide our judgements and facilitate a person-centred humanised approach.

Empathic knowledge in care (Galvin and Todres, 2010)

Galvin and Todres (2010) recognised along with many other psychologist and care practitioners that an empathetic understanding of the other person could help facilitate person-centred care. Through their philosophical explorations they established that empathetic knowledge of the other person could be developed through embodied relational understanding, explained in the previous section. Intrinsic to embodied relational understanding is embodied interpretation which can provide evidence for the use of head, heart and hands in care. This is achieved through:

- Being present to the stories of the other person
- Entering into developing meanings
- Dwelling with and holding the other person
- Finding words for the 'fuzzy' 'felt' sense of embodied dwelling which Gendlin (1962, 1992) identified as 'felt sense'

An understanding of insiderness through embodied relational understanding and empathetic knowledge can facilitate ensuring that a person's humanity is respected.

Dwelling mobility

Since the development of the Humanising Values Framework, Todres and Galvin have continued to develop an understanding of well-being based on the developing philosophical and psychological phenomenology; as part of this they explored dwelling and mobility.

For Todres and Galvin (2010; Galvin and Todres, 2011), dwelling and mobility are bipolar constructs with neither pole being negative or positive. The person can have a sense of well-being whether they are dwelling or mobile – both are seen as necessary for the person. Their writing was founded on the earlier work of Heidegger, who identified that people who had a sense of well-being were experiencing a 'felt-sense' of homelike being in the world (Figure 5.2).

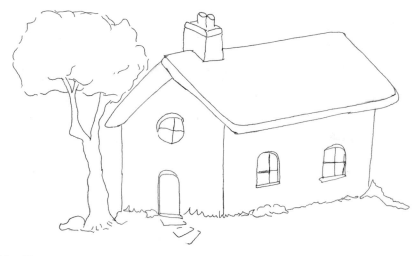

Figure 5.2   Home

Heidegger expressed this with the terms of spatiality, temporality, intersubjectivity, mood, personal identity and embodiments, which are all components of being in the world. He offered the examples of adventure and being at home, rootedness and flow, peace and possibility to facilitate understanding. Todres and Galvin called this 'dwelling mobility'. They identified how dwelling and mobility were experienced in each of Heidegger's ways of experiencing the world (see Table 5.2).

Table 5.2　Todres and Galvin: types of dwelling mobility

Mode	Dwelling	Mobility
Spatial	Being at home	Sense of adventure
Temporal	Grounded in moment	Forward movement
Intersubjective	Kinship and belonging	Mysterious attraction
Mood	Peace	Excitement/desire
Personal identity	Being at one with the world	'I can do this'
Embodied	Comfort	Vitality

Person-centred approaches have developed from existential and phenomenological philosophy and humanistic psychology, as can be seen in the work of Todres and Galvin; this areas is still growing and developing. Our understanding of well-being and how to support a sense of well-being is increasing, and given some of the research into person-centred compassion outlined in Chapter 4, we can see its significance in care becoming more established.

Chapter summary

This chapter has focused on the development of psychology of person-centred approaches and the underlying philosophies of this. The genealogy of philosophy was described, along with how that related to the genesis and continued metamorphosis of the schools of psychology. It was established that all the early schools of psychology had an influence on humanistic psychology, which was the foundation of person-centred approaches. The chapter concluded with an explanation of new understandings of this approach from contemporary philosophers and psychologists recognising how together they offer greater insight.

Further study

The Health Foundation has a new web-based resource for person-centred care, where you can access and read materials that are relevant for you if you are a formal or informal carer or a service user. There is the opportunity to sign up for email alerts for any new things occurring and hear about how others are implementing person-centred care. See: http://personcentredcare.health.org.uk/

Activity outline answers

Activity 5.3   Critical thinking

Read the case study of Agatha Wright. How would you describe her personality? What do you think has influenced this?

Your understanding of Agatha will depend on your personal worldview, but as explained in the following text a simple reading of the story will lead you to think that what is important for Agatha is her relationships with other people, particularly her family. Her father and husband appear to have a significant impact on her feelings and behaviour.

If we consider her well-being from a humanistic perspective, we might see her as receiving the unconditional positive regard she needed until her uncle died and after that she only received positive regard through 'conditions of worth'. She only experienced positive regard when she did something to please others. She talks about being happy and having special moments like being smiled at, kissed and touched by loved ones; therefore she is not purely responding to conditions of worth and her self-esteem may be quite high.

Activity 5.4   Critical thinking

After you read Matthew's story, identify the significant factors that you will need to take into consideration when caring for him.

A simple reading of Matthew's story would lead us to believe that independence and achievements are important to him. Therefore, if you were to be caring for him, it is highly important that he is enabled to be as independent as possible, that his agency is supported and that he is facilitated to make his own decisions. It will also be important to highlight what he is able to achieve and his strengths.

Activity 5.5   Critical thinking

In mental healthcare, some people are described as 'not being in touch with reality', as they are diagnosed with an illness that means they are experiencing delusions. Look at the list below and decide which of these thoughts might be delusional:

I have an angel that looks after me

I have conversations with God

I am more intelligent than you

I have a sixth sense: I know when something bad is going to happen

I am famous

I am a disgusting person

All of these statements may be delusional but they may also have some validity; there may be some evidence to support them. To be person-centred, we need to accept other people's sense of reality but we also need to be congruent so that we do not agree that these statements are true; however, we do need to recognise that they are part of their reality. As carers, what is important is the impact these thoughts have on the person. If they are increasing their well-being, there may be no necessity for us to do anything other than validate that that is what they think, but if they are making the person unwell we may need to intervene.

References

American Psychological Society (2015) *About APA and about Psychology*. Available at: www.apa.org/support/about/apa/psychology.aspx#answer (accessed September 2015).

Barker, S. (2007) *Vital Notes for Nurses: Psychology*. Oxford: Blackwell.

Barker, S. (2011) *Midwives' Emotional Care of Women becoming Mothers*. Newcastle Upon Tyne: Cambridge Scholars Publishing.

British Psychological Society (2013) *Good Dementia Care*. Available at: www.bps.org.uk/news/psychology-integral-good-dementia-care (accessed September 2015).

British Psychological Society (BPS) (2015) *Psychology*. Available at: www.bps.org.uk/ (accessed April 2015).

Carlson, N.R., Martin, G.N. and Buskist, W. (2004) *Psychology*, 2nd edn. London: Pearson.

Galvin, K. and Todres, L. (2010) 'Research-based empathic knowledge for nursing: A translational strategy for disseminating phenomenological research findings to provide evidence for caring practice', *International Journal of Nursing Studies*, 48: 522–30.

Galvin, K. and Todres, L. (2011) 'Kinds of well-being: A conceptual framework that provides direction for caring', *International Journal of Qualitative Studies on Health Well-being*, 6 (4): 10362.

Galvin, K. and Todres, L. (2013) *Caring and Well-Being: A Lifeworld Approach*. London: Routledge.

Gendlin, E.T. (1962) *Experiencing and the Creation of Meaning*. Glencoe, NY: Free Press.

Gendlin, E.T. (1992) 'The primacy of the body, not the primacy of perception: How the body knows the situation and philosophy', *Man and World*, 25 (3–4): 341–53. Available at: www.focusing.org/pdf/primacy_excerpt.pdf (accessed September 2015).

Gerrig, R.J., Zimbardo, P.G., Svartdal, F., Brennen, T., Donaldson, R. and Archer, T. (2012) *Psychology and Life*. Harlow: Pearson.

Gross, R. (2005) *Psychology: The Science of Mind and Behaviour*, 5th edn. London: Hodder Arnold.

Health Care Professions Council (HCPC) (2015) *Person-Centred Care*. Available at: www.hpc-uk.org/publications/research/index.asp?id=668 (accessed September 2015).

Health Foundation (2014) *Person-Centred Care Made Simple*. Available at: www.health.org.uk/sites/default/files/PersonCentredCareMadeSimple.pdf (accessed September 2015).

James, W. (1890) *The Principles of Psychology*. Available at: https://archive.org/stream/theprinciplesofp01jameuoft#page/n11/mode/2up (accessed September 2015).

Kitwood, T. (1997) *Dementia Reconsidered: The Person Comes First*. Maidenhead: Open University Press.

MacKinlay, E.B. (2001) 'The spiritual dimension of caring: Applying a model for spiritual tasks of aging', *Journal of Religious Gerontology*, 12 (3–4): 151–66.

MacKinlay, E. (2011) 'Creative processes to bring out expressions of spirituality: Working with people who have dementia', in H. Lee and T. Adams (eds), *Creative Approaches in Dementia Care*. Basingstoke: Palgrave Macmillan, pp. 212–29.

Morrissey, J. and Callaghan, P. (2011) *Communication Skills for Mental Health Nurses*. Maidenhead: Open University Press, McGraw-Hill Education.

Morse, J.M., Bottorff, J., Anderson, G., O'Brien, B. and Solberg, S. (1992) 'Beyond empathy: Expanding expressions of caring', *Journal of Advanced Nursing*, 17: 809–21.

Robinson, D.K. (2010) 'Gustav Fechner: 150 years of Elemente der Psychophysik', *History of Psychology*, 13 (4): 409–10.

Rogers, C.R. (1961) *A Therapist's View of Psychotherapy: On Becoming a Person*. London: Constable.

Royal College of Nursing (RCN) (2015) *Person-Centred Care*. Available at: www.rcn.org.uk/development/practice/cpd_online_learning/dignity_in_health_care/person-centred_care (accessed September 2015).

Todres, L. (2007) *Embodied Enquiry: Phenomenological Touchstones for Research, Psychotherapy and Spirituality*. Basingstoke: Palgrave Macmillan.

Todres, L. (2008) 'Being with that: The relevance of embodied understanding in practice', *Qualitative Health Research*, 8 (11): 1566–73.

Todres, L. and Galvin, K. (2010) '"Dwelling-mobility": An existential theory of well-being', *International Journal of Qualitative Studies on Health and Well-being*, 5: 5444.

Todres, L., Galvin, K. and Dahlberg, K. (2014) '"Caring for insiderness": Phenomenologically informed insights that can guide practice', *International Journal of Qualitative Studies on Health and Well-being*, 9: 21421.

Todres, L., Galvin, K.T. and Holloway, I. (2009) 'The humanization of healthcare: A value framework for qualitative research', *International Journal of Qualitative Studies on Health and Well-being*, 4: 66–77.

Verity, J. and Lee, H. (2011) 'Reigniting the human spirit', in H. Lee and T. Adams (eds), *Creative Approaches in Dementia Care*. Basingstoke: Palgrave Macmillan, pp. 16–32.

6 The Care Practitioner

Sue Barker and Gareth Morgan

Who am I to provide your care?

Of what am I to be aware?

Do I talk and of myself share?

Am I silent beneath your glare?

Do I hold you – Do I dare?

Or will I be found wanting there?

Who am I to provide your care?

We move as one, we are a pair.

Learning objectives

Most people have an opinion on who should be a care practitioner, with many children being told in childhood that they would make a good nurse or doctor. How accurate are these assertions? Is there a particular type of person who should be a care practitioner? This chapter's learning objectives are to:

- Describe how different psychologists explain personality
- Define self-concept and self-esteem
- Identify explanations of motivation, perception and attribution
- Recognise professional issues in the use of **self-disclosure**

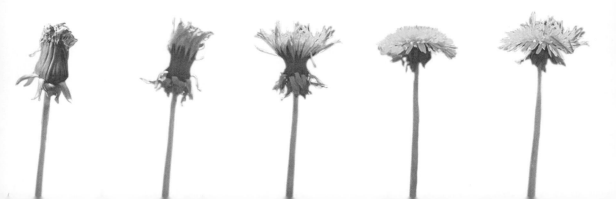

> ## Activity 6.1   Critical thinking
>
> When you were young, did your family say that they could see you becoming a firefighter, farmer, doctor, nanny? If they did, why did they suggest this?
>
> *An outline answer can be found at the end of the chapter.*

Introduction

The previous chapters in this book are a journey starting from exploring the major theoretical perspectives in psychology and how psychologists develop their understanding. In Chapter 2, this basic understanding led to an exploration of health, well-being and illness through the lifespan. Chapter 3 considered suffering: the loss of well-being and the underpinning reason for the need of compassionate care. Chapter 4 went on to discover what compassionate care is through the models available and the culture in which it is provided. Chapter 5 explored compassion and compassionate care at a deeper philosophical and psychological level through an understanding of person-centred care.

This chapter explores the character of the care practitioner through mostly scientific psychological theory and research. It is important that care practitioners are aware of the empirical scientific explanation of themselves and their role if they are to move from a biomedical approach to a person-centred approach. This chapter offers an examination of care practitioners through theoretical explanations of personality, self-awareness and self-concept. It explores how caregivers feel, their self-esteem and how they behave, through mostly cognitive theories of perception, motivation, attitude and attribution. Cognitive theorists have had a big impact on understanding individual differences to explain behaviour and psychological therapies adopted into health and social care services.

The chapter starts by defining and describing personality as it can be seen as an overarching concept. This is followed by a more detailed consideration of psychological explanations of individual differences between people. Personality is a broad concept and has been theorised in all the psychological perspectives.

Historically, care has been regarded as an activity undertaken by women as part of their other established roles such as mother, daughter or wife, with little status or monetary remuneration. The underlying socio-cultural context and prevailing system of political power within a society influence the status and stereotypes held in regard of its citizens such as care practitioners: the cultural hegemony.

Regardless of cultural stereotypes, care practitioners can be as diverse in **character** and **temperament** as those they help. Their status and salary can be very low or above the average wage as can their educational achievements and attainments within contemporary cultures. Despite this diversity, it remains important to understand ourselves and each other if we are to work to our best ability and provide the highest-quality care (see Chapters 7 and 9).

The overarching concept that brings together an understanding of the person, in this case the care practitioner, is called 'personality'. Unsurprisingly, psychology offers a number of definitions and theories through which to understand this concept, including the individual characteristics encompassed by it. Whilst the different psychological perspectives identify personality in a number of ways such as a structure or a process, a broad definition will offer two working hypotheses through which to undertake a more detailed exploration.

A cognitive and scientific psychological definition of personality could be:

The relatively stable traits or characteristics demonstrated by a person over a period of time and in different situations.

A more humanistic, person-centred psychological definition of personality could be:

The interaction between an individual's 'felt sense' (which provides meaning through embodied relational knowing) and the world in which the person lives.

Activity 6.2   Critical thinking

- How would you describe your personality?
- Do you describe it in terms of feeling? Likes, dislikes?
- Do you describe it in terms of abilities?
- Do you describe it in terms of what you do?
- Who am I and what gives meaning to my life?

An outline answer can be found at the end of the chapter.

Personality theories

Psychodynamic

This theoretical perspective is based on the psychodynamic theory of Freud. Freud is considered to be one of the great thinkers of the twentieth century. He was a Viennese physician who fled to England to escape the Nazi occupation of Austria. Freud was influenced by the prevailing socio-political environment of his time but he still has something to offer the care practitioners and psychologists of today (see Chapters 1 and 2).

The term 'psychodynamic' implies that active forces within the personality motivate behaviour particularly between the three component parts of the personality or psyche. These three component parts are the id, ego and superego. The id and the superego are largely unconscious and the ego is largely conscious (with some preconscious and unconscious components). As with an iceberg, most of the personality lies beneath the surface and therefore cannot be seen (see Figure 1.2).

Within Freud's theory, he describes stages of psychosexual development to attaining an adult personality. If a person has problems successfully moving through the three early psychosexual stages, their development may be arrested (fixation), they may return to that stage at times of adult stress (regression) or they may develop an ongoing personality type linked to that stage. Freud's stages of psychosexual development are discussed in Chapter 2, along with their impact on adult personality.

Freud offers care practitioners the understanding that their personality is **dynamic**: it is always in the process of changing and there are some parts of themselves they will never be able to know (they are unconscious). Also, their personality is perpetually in conflict: there is always a conflict between the id and superego which is being balanced by the ego. To gain increased self-awareness and understanding of themselves, according to psychodynamic theorists, people can go through analysis with a therapist (see Chapter 7).

Behavioural and cognitive theories

In contrast to the psychodynamic theorists, behaviourists suggest that babies are born solely with the ability to learn (see Chapters 1 and 2). They explain that all that can be known of a person is their observed individual behaviour, which is developed through their environment – it is a person's behaviour that determines their personality. Personality, individual characteristics and apparent traits, therefore, are learned in the same way as any other behaviour.

Whilst people on the whole learn according to classical and operant conditioning, some behaviours that appear to be novel occur which led to the **cognitive shift**. Bandura's (1965) social learning theory (see Chapter 1) appeared to offer some explanation for this with his vicarious learning, although this does not fully account for novel behaviour.

Bandura, whilst accepting the learning processes of classical and operant conditioning, identified through his studies, including the widely disseminated **Bobo doll experiments** in 1965, people learned through observation and imitation as well. This ability was greatly increased through effective role models. Effective role models are those who are socially accepted, rewarded and similar in some way to the observer. With these characteristics the role models were more likely to be imitated, for example both having a caring occupation.

Bobo doll experiment

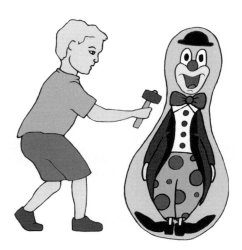

In 1961 and 1963, Albert Bandura developed some empirical experiments to test his theory that children learn behaviour such as aggression. He set up experiments where children were observed playing with a number of toys, including a 'bobo doll', an inflatable doll weighted at the bottom so that when knocked it does not fall over. When children were given a bobo doll to play with, they did not undertake any aggressive play, but after they had observed an adult (role model) being aggressive towards the doll, they **imitated** this behaviour (Figure 6.1).

These experiments have been criticised, as would be expected for any experimental design. It was suggested that all that was observed was the children imitating the

Figure 6.1   Boy hitting a bobo doll

adults' behaviour, and not that they were being aggressive. It has also been identified that there might be a number of reasons for this, such as attempts to please the experimenter.

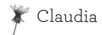

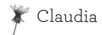 Claudia

Claudia is a student nurse. She is 40 years old and had always wanted to be a nurse, but she became pregnant as a teenager and did not complete her secondary education. Her children are now independent and successful in their career paths. Claudia's daughter encouraged her to realise her ambition. With support from her family and staff at the local college she attended, she was successful on the health and social care programme and gained a place at university.

Claudia is liked by her peers. They see her as warm and friendly and people talk to her when they are struggling. Claudia appears to be a 'mother figure' to her much younger study group. The tutors at the university and her clinical mentor demonstrate acknowledgment and appreciation of this by telling her how much she is helping the other students. Sometimes this is difficult for Claudia as she too struggles with the academic work and has to manage not only her own time but that of her family as well. Taking responsibility for what appears to her to be everyone has left her feeling stressed. This has led to her 'comfort eating' and recent weight gain.

This theory outlines that through a process of observation and imitation called **modelling** children develop their self-concept and self-efficacy, which is strengthened by continued learning in adulthood. In the case study of Claudia, we can see that she had a limited education and felt unable to realise her ambition of becoming a nurse. Her self-efficacy could be identified as low, which may have led to a low self-esteem as well. This may have been learned in her childhood and then reinforced through adolescence.

- *Self-concept*: A collection of thoughts or ideas about oneself; for example, 'I am a caring person'
- *Self-efficacy*: The belief in one's own ability to achieve a goal; for example, 'I am able to dress a wound'

Whilst this is rather simplistic, it does allow recognition that a person's early experiences and their environment can have a dramatic impact on their later perceived personality. Also using this theory, we can see that despite Claudia's struggle with the academic work, she is acknowledged as a role model for the other students by her tutors and mentor. This is being reinforced (rewarded) by the tutors and mentor through their praise of her, which encourages her to continue this behaviour.

This theory has been influential in education as care practitioners are usually encouraged to develop through watching and copying effective role models usually identified as mentors. Modelling, according to this theory, facilitates the care practitioner's adoption of attitudes, values and also the ability to **self-evaluate**.

The ability to self-evaluate their behaviours including attitudes and values increases the individual's ability to function within society. Self-evaluation can be seen as closely linked to self-awareness, which is recognised as an essential skill for care practitioners (see Chapter 7).

Trait theories

Two theories of personality have been outlined above: psychodynamic and social learning theory. These are considered to be **process** personality theories. There are also structural theories of personality such as **trait** theories. Structural theories of personality identify personality as fixed and in most cases something a person is born with. This undervalues the influence of environment and psychological processes. Traits or individual temperament are considered to be biological or genetic theories of personality:

- *Temperament*: The natural disposition of the person, which may include their mental, emotional and physical attributes
- *Traits*: Stable sources of individual differences that characterise what a person is like

Hans Eysenck (1916–97) identified that the personality embraces just three major traits: **extroversion, neuroticism** and **psychoticism**. These are continuums with people having differing amounts of each and therefore at different points along a pole of, for example, extreme extroversion to extreme **introversion**:

- *Extroversion*: The extent to which a person engages with other people; an extrovert is said to continuously seek the company of others. The other extreme of this polemic trait is introversion, which occurs in people who prefer their own company to that of others
- *Neuroticism*: Relates to how much a person worries or is anxious. They could have high anxiety levels and therefore have a high level of neuroticism, which is one extreme of the pole. A person who is more philosophical possesses little of this trait: the other end of the pole
- *Psychoticism*: Refers to how well a person 'fits' in with their culture. If the person exhibits high levels of psychoticism they may be considered **deviant,** for example by not following social rules about acceptable behaviour. Having extremely low levels of psychoticism, the other end of the pole, the person may be over-compliant and a rule-follower but they may also be considered to have no personality

If we consider the case study of Claudia again, we can make some assumptions based on her behaviour about where she is on the three personality-traits poles identified by Eysenck. Claudia appears to enjoy the company of others, given her relationships being warm and friendly with the other students, and her desire to nurse could lead us to believe that she is nearer the polarity of extroversion rather than introversion. She is recognised as a good example for the other students and is doing well on her course; therefore she is likely to have low psychoticism. Claudia may be nearer the polarity of neuroticism than the opposing philosophical state, given her concern about achieving her ambition and her current level of stress.

Eysenck gives clear biological explanations for extroversion and neuroticism but his biological explanation for psychoticism is limited. Extroversion and neuroticism have been linked to the **limbic system** and **reticular formation** in the brain stem whereas psychoticism has been linked to the **dopaminergic** (neurotransmitter) system.

Activity 6.3   Reflection

Take a few minutes to consider if all the different people you have met have personalities that can be explained by using these three traits.

As this is a reflection, there is no outline answer at the end of the chapter.

Eysenck's traits have been considered limited and have been expanded by subsequent psychologists to the 'big five' traits: neuroticism, extroversion, openness to experience, agreeableness and conscientiousness. Whilst these are useful to undertake empirical research, any theory that limits understanding of a person to 3, 5 or even 10 traits appears to limit our understanding of humanity and the need for individualised person-centred care.

The above theories offer a structural understanding of personality (trait) with internal mechanisms based on genetics and a process-orientated theory (behaviourism) which offers an environmental understanding of personality. The humanists, particularly Rogers (1951, 1961), avoid both of these approaches as they find them unhelpful in understanding the individual. The humanists could be described as incorporating a spiritual element into the structure and processes of personality already identified.

Humanistic

Self-concept is central to Rogers' (1951, 1961) theory but his explanation of self-concept differs from the cognitive understanding (social learning theory above). His self-concept is based on the individual's phenomenological field. This is their subjective experiences of the world, which is always changing; it is fluid. The person's world (phenomenological field) is their perception of their experiences. These perceptions or their perceptual field provides the individual's sense of reality; it is their own personal **reality**. This reality is the only reality available to the person (see Chapters 1 and 5). Rogers does not accept that the person is a victim to their genetic make-up or environmental conditions but that these come together as part of the person's phenomenological field which is subjectively perceived by them.

The individual's emotions, values and beliefs are significant factors in their perception of their life world – the phenomenological field. The person may experience a sense of themselves when all their sensory and visceral experiences can be assimilated but at the same time are open to change. Rogers writes that a person needs to 'open their spirit' to all of life's possibilities: the possibility of experiencing the rich tapestry of emotions and existential being.

For a person to be open to their experiences and to have an optimistic view of themselves and the world, they need to receive **non-judgemental positive regard** (see Chapters 1, 2, 5 and 7). Receiving positive regard allows the person to fully realise who they are and for their perception of their ideal self and actual self to be close together. This results in high self-esteem and self-awareness, with the opportunity for the person to fully experience the world and realise their potential.

Summary

This section has considered the differing personality theories from each psychological perspective. Trait theorists and psychodynamic theorists offer a structural explanation of the personality whereas behavioural and cognitive theorists offer a process-orientated explanation. Unlike trait theories psychodynamic, behavioural and cognitive theories all allow for development and change. Trait theories only allow for change if there is an underlying biological disturbance such as disease or trauma, whereas Rogers offers a fluid, subjective sense of self related to life world experiences both internal and external to the individual.

To explore the personality of the care practitioner in more detail and to gain an understanding of the individuals they share care with, a good starting point is the understanding they have of themselves. Self-awareness is a crucial skill for care practitioners (see Chapter 7), so the importance of self-esteem will next be considered and then an exploration of what motivates an individual's behaviour and how care practitioners develop their understanding of other people's behaviour.

Self-awareness

Self-awareness is considered an essential skill for all care practitioners; indeed for many therapies the aim is to develop self-awareness and self-acceptance (see Chapter 7). To be self-aware is to be able to bring to consciousness all of our experiences: to experience ourselves as being different and separate from others at the same time as being in relationship with them. It is about understanding ourselves and our thoughts, feelings and behaviours (Table 6.1).

Table 6.1 Methods and concepts in self-awareness

Method for developing self-awareness	Concepts related to self-awareness
Meditating	Thoughts, feelings, behaviour
Reflection	Beliefs, attitudes, values
Mindfulness	Hopes and fears
Gaining feedback from others	Likes and dislikes
Comparing oneself to others	Past experiences
Comparing oneself to professional ethics or religious teaching	Past relationships
Psychological therapy	Traumatic events

Activity 6.4   Reflection

Take a few minutes to consider recent feedback that you were given by a mentor, carer or person you were giving care to.

- Is this feedback accurate?
- What evidence was this judgement based on?

As this is a reflection, there is no outline answer at the end of the chapter.

Self-esteem

Self-esteem is an important concept in humanistic psychology as the two earliest theorists in this area, Maslow (1954) and Rogers (1951), both identified people's need to have self-esteem. Self-esteem is the feeling we have about ourselves: self-worth. Maslow identified esteem as a deficiency drive, highlighting that people need esteem to remain well. There are two types of esteem according to him: self-esteem and esteem from being valued and respected by others. People with high self-esteem have greater self-worth and confidence. They can also be more productive and competent.

Significantly, Rogers suggested the lack of self-esteem as being a root cause for psychological discomfort. He stated that people who are struggling tend to deride themselves, which interferes with their ability to accept who they are and reach their potential. His therapeutic work allows people to engage their motivational drives and reach their potential.

Motivation

Motivation is a significant area of individual differences examined by psychologists and can be seen to be an important factor in achievement of personal goals/potential. Motivation is understood and explained in different ways, depending on the psychological perspective. Some psychologists define motivation as an impulse, desire or need that leads to action, whilst others define it as the energising force of behaviour.

For humanistic psychologists, motivation can be seen as internal and individual to the person (see Chapter 1).

Abraham Maslow (1908–70)

Maslow was said to be the first of the humanist psychologists. He developed a hierarchy of needs, which can offer a framework for exploring motivation (see Chapter 1 and Figure 1.5). Maslow's hierarchy of needs places the most basic or essential needs at the bottom of his pyramid and indicates that people must work their way from the bottom to the top of the hierarchy. They achieve this movement through two different drives (motivations), and these drives or actions are to achieve what the person needs. The two drives are called **deficiency drives** or motives and **growth drives** or motives:

- Deficiency motives are those lowest in the hierarchy: physiological needs, safety, love, belonging and esteem needs
- Growth motives are those at the top of the hierarchy and promote self-actualisation: cognitive needs, aesthetic needs and self-actualisation

Deficiency motives or drives

These drives or motives lead people to fulfil basic or essential needs. If one of these needs were unfilled, the person may become injured or ill, but if the need were fulfilled or restored it could reduce the risk of harm to the person. These deficiency drives are always active, and they continuously exert pressure as physiological needs such as thirst and hunger can only be **satiated** for a short period of time.

Growth motives

These motives or drives lead the person to enrich and expand their experiences or phenomenological field. They address a sense of curiosity, creativeness and ambition.

Biopsychologists

In contrast to the humanistic theory of motivation (which acknowledges a biological element) are the biopsychological theories of motivation. One of the biological theories of motivation is the homeostatic drive, which describes the maintenance of the internal functioning of the body. Homeostasis is derived from the Greek language *homo* meaning 'same' and *stasis* meaning 'stoppage'. *Drive* is generally considered to mean 'propel, force or push'. Therefore, this theory explains the force to maintain or stop a process or movement. This is a **homogenous** theory: one that indicates how all people are similar.

The homeostatic drive:

- Refers to the internal body processes which work together to maintain a constant optimal bodily environment
- If the body's temperature becomes higher than is optimal an imbalance will occur and the body will respond to restore its equilibrium
- Regulates, for example, blood pressure, heart rate, digestion, respiration

There are a number of biological processes that facilitate the body remaining within certain parameters. The body 'needs' certain conditions in order to function and these needs lead to 'action', hence 'motivation'. In the case of the body's need for oxygen, the diaphragm muscle pulls down into the abdomen, the chest expands and air rushes into the lungs. There is a gaseous exchange in the lungs, transporting oxygen to the blood, which is circulated by the heart. This is a basic biological motivation but the need for homeostasis can be seen in other actions that are considered more psychological such as the **fight-or-flight response**.

Fight-or-flight response

This is sometimes referred to as the 'fight, flight or freeze response'. It is where an acute stress reaction has been triggered by a feared situation (perception). This trigger sets off a biological process called the 'hypothalamic–pituitary–adrenal axis' (HPA axis), and is highlighted in Figure 3.2. This provides the motivation for the person to run away or to fight in order to restore homeostasis (Figure 6.2).

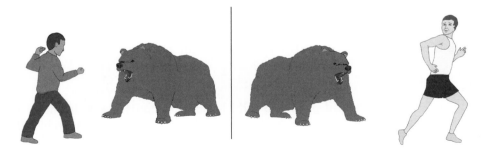

Figure 6.2   Fight or flight

Psychodynamic

The psychodynamic perspective offers an instinct theory of motivation. Freud initially identified libido as the motivating force for behaviour that is innate: all people are born with it, so, whilst his explanation of it is psychodynamic, the force is biological. This force is found in the id, the pleasure-seeking part of the psyche or mind. This innate drive is in conflict with the learned morality of the superego (see Chapter 1). Freud later in his life distinguished between two motivational forces: the libido (sexuality) part of the life instinct or Eros; and the death instinct, which he called Thanos. This represented an inborn destructiveness which could reduce inner tension. He also outlines that Thanos is leading the person back to the peace or lack of conflict found by the baby in the womb and which can only be found once again in death.

Whilst the instinctual drive identifies the homogeneity of people, it does allow for some individual differences in behaviour.

Social learning theory

As already established, social learning theory developed from behaviourism and was part of the cognitive shift, and this theory of motivation is in direct opposition to the biological (nature) ones: it offers environmental (nurture) explanations. It is therefore based on association, reinforcement (rewards) and modelling. Social learning theory offers two sets of motivators or drives, both of which have been developed through modelling (see above):

- *Intrinsic*: This is where motivation comes from within the person and its fulfilment. It is where the person gains rewards for their behaviour from within themselves, for example assisting with a patient's personal hygiene, leaving the care practitioner with a feeling of pleasure
- *Extrinsic*: This is where the motivation to enact behaviour comes from outside the person. For a care practitioner, this could be where they are induced to perform a task by the offer of money

Internal motivators have been seen to be longer-lasting than external motivators, as when the external motivator is removed, for example the person is no longer paid, the behaviour is **extinguished**: it stops. To develop internal motivation is considered to result in greater commitment or improved performance.

 Mel

Chris is a 50-year-old occupational therapist in an assertive outreach team in a large northern city. Chris is currently working with a range of clients, one of whom, Mel, recently left the care of the inpatient service and is now living in a social housing flat in a deprived part of the city. Mel's condition has greatly impacted on her capacity to undertake her preferred occupations. Mel wants to commence work in a charity shop ahead of a move into the retail sector.

Case study

(Continued)

(Continued)

As an occupational therapist, Chris is keen to engage Mel in her preferred occupations but is conscious of Mel's problems with time-keeping and engaging with the caring services – much of Mel's week is spent at home sleeping and watching daytime television whilst gorging on junk food. Chris often calls at the house but is unable to affect an entry as Mel is either sleeping or reluctant to answer the door.

Chris feels that this case is typical of so many that he has faced in recent years. He feels disillusioned with his calling because one of the tenets of the profession is to engage clients actively in their occupations. However, engaging with people in a meaningful manner seems an aspiration that is ethically laudable but seems out of touch with the reality of occupational therapy on the ground.

If we consider the case study of Mel, we can see that Chris is becoming disillusioned. He has learned that to support meaningful activity is important for a person's sense of well-being but his current learning is that this is unachievable. His self-efficacy is low due to the absence of any internal or external motivators or reinforcements: despite his efforts, Mel is not engaging.

Summary

Cognitive and social learning theories of motivation identify that it is something that is developed through nurture, whereas the biological and psychodynamic theories provide nature explanations. Maslow's theory can be considered to accept both a nature and nurture basis for motivation, but both he and Rogers suggest that there is more to the person and that their needs have a spiritual component, too, which the other theories do not recognise.

Motivation and locus of control

A concept linked to motivation and self-efficacy is the **locus of control** – *locus* meaning 'place' or 'location' and 'locus of control' meaning 'where control is situated or stems from'. The premise is that if the person has an internal locus of control, they are more likely to have high self-efficacy and be more likely to enact desired behaviour: they are motivated to initiate action. This is different to the intrinsic and extrinsic motivators discussed above. The motivators above are indicating where the reward reinforcing the behaviour to maintain it comes from, whereas the locus of control identifies who or what has the control or power to initiate the behaviour. If we return to the case study of Mel, we can see that for Chris there were no rewards whether internal or external, resulting in low self-efficacy. Low self-efficacy can lead to low self-esteem and create psychological distress, according to the humanistic psychologists. How Chris manages this will partly depend on his locus of control: where he thinks the power is based.

Julian B. Rotter (1916–2014) developed the concept of the locus of control as part of his social learning theory approach to personality, behaviour and motivation, therefore focused on nurture theories. He identified one personality characteristic that influenced behaviour was whether the person had an internal or external locus of control. These characteristics are not traits as per Eysenck's theory, a nature theory: they can and will change through the principles of behaviourism such as reinforcement.

A person with an internal locus of control would identify that they had control of their behaviour, health and lifestyle. A person with an external locus of control would identify the control of their behaviour and their experiences as being external to themselves. External controls could include the government, their parents, their partner, their **manager** or God. Another form of external control is where there is no power base or control and their behaviour and experiences are believed to be according to chance.

For Chris, if he has an internal locus of control, he may believe that as Mel is not engaging he needs to work harder or attempt a different approach. He may seek guidance from colleagues or supervisors and search recent research evidence. If, on the other hand, Chris has an external locus of control, he will see powerful others or chance as the reason for the lack of engagement. If he identified Mel as having the power to make the changes, he will blame her for the lack of progress – which in turn will affect their relationship. If he believes that it is due to chance or fate, he may just resign himself to the situation and not make any changes.

Locus of control is seen as one of four core ways in which people undertake a self-evaluation. The four core self-evaluations are locus of control, neuroticism, self-efficacy and self-esteem. Internal locus of control, low neuroticism, high self-efficacy and high self-esteem are considered to result in high job satisfaction and achievements. We can see that for Chris, he is disillusioned, which could indicate his low self-efficacy, low self-esteem and external locus of control.

Summary

The psychological theories of motivation that have been considered have indicated that care practitioners and those they care for can be motivated by their biological, psychological, social and spiritual needs. How they respond to the initial motivation and whether motivated behaviour continues will in part be determined by the responses they received and whether their needs are fulfilled.

Theories of motivation, particularly the nurture ones, will be influenced by the person's perception of their own bodies and the environment in which they are developing. It is therefore important that we consider the theories of perception but it is also important to recognise that these theories are biological (nature), cognitive (nurture) or gestalt (pattern recognition).

Perception

In psychology there are two distinct areas of research related to perception. They are generally called 'object perception/sensory perception' and 'person perception/social perception'. Both types of perception, however, have features in common:

- *Selection*: Focusing on a particular object or part of a person's behaviour
- *Organisation*: Trying to gain an understanding of the complete object or person
- *Inference*: Making assumptions about the object or person without direct perceptual information

Object perception

There are a number of psychological theories about how people perceive objects and why they get it wrong at times. These have developed through studies in the cognitive perspective, and cognitive researchers have tried to understand how information from the senses is received, processed, stored and retrieved. There are four major approaches to this:

- Bottom up
- Top down
- Cyclic
- Gestalt

Object perception theories

Bottom up
This theory was developed by Gibson (1966) and is called the 'theory of direct perception'. His research was mainly in the area of visual perception and he suggested that there was no need for inferences because there was enough unambiguous information in the environment for people to perceive an object.

Top down
Gregory (1966) theorised that perceptions are **unconscious inferences** and developed a **constructivist** theory. He indicated that people already have an idea of what objects they are going to find in their mind and they then check the environment for these objects – this is called a **perceptual hypothesis**. It can lead to **illusions** where a person finds what they expect to see, rather than what is there. He also suggested that people look for **perceptual constancy**. An example of a perceptual constancy is that if something is farther away it is smaller.

Cyclic
Neisser's (1976) 'cyclic model of perception' offers a top-down and bottom-up theory. It is a process where the mind is actively searching the environment for evidence which offers a rich source of information.

Gestalt object perceptual theory

Gregory's theory focused on inferences (ideas or hypotheses), a top-down approach, and Gibson's theory focused on the detail, a bottom-up approach; the gestalt approach focuses on organisation. The gestalt theorists identified that people focus on wholes rather than on isolated sensations. They offer a number of laws by which people adopt a best-fit approach to perceiving objects (see Figure 6.3):

- *Proximity*: If items are close together, they are seen as a whole
- *Similarity*: Things that are similar to each other are grouped together
- *Continuity*: People tend to look for continuity of items, rather than separate items
- *Closure*: When parts of what appears to be an object are missing, they are not noticed
- *Part–whole relationships*: Sense will be made of an overall picture, rather than sense being made of the smaller parts

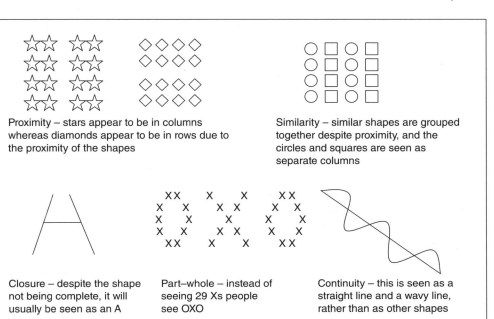

Proximity – stars appear to be in columns whereas diamonds appear to be in rows due to the proximity of the shapes

Similarity – similar shapes are grouped together despite proximity, and the circles and squares are seen as separate columns

Closure – despite the shape not being complete, it will usually be seen as an A

Part–whole – instead of seeing 29 Xs people see OXO

Continuity – this is seen as a straight line and a wavy line, rather than as other shapes

Figure 6.3 Gestalt principles

Illusions

Top-down theories and gestalt theories offer explanations for illusions. There are illusions to be found in all of the senses but most well-known are visual illusions and these fall into four types:

- *Distortions*: Misperceived objects (examples: the optical illusion works of Franz Carl Müller-Lyer, Mario Ponzo and Mark Titchener)
- *Ambiguous figures*: Same visual sensory input but different perceptions (examples: Rubin's vase, Leeper's woman)
- *Paradoxical figures*: False assumptions (examples: Penrose impossible objects, Escher's pictures)
- *Fictions*: Seeing what is not there (example: Kanizsa triangle)

Illusions are difficult to explain unless there is mental processing of sensory information in object perception.

Social perception

Social perception involves more than recognising objects; it is about how we understand our social world. This can have an impact on self-awareness, self-efficacy, self-esteem, psychological well-being and relationships. All the psychological perspective can offer an interpretation of our behaviour in social settings based on their underlying principles (outlined in Chapter 1). The term 'social perception' has been used most widely by cognitive and behavioural theorists, so most of the theories are from this genre.

In social perception, as well as cognitive perceptual illusions, what we 'see' might not always be correct.

Cognitive perspective within social perception

There are four models of the thinking person within social perception:

- *Consistency seekers*: This is where the person seeks to reduce inconsistencies in thoughts about the social world as inconsistency causes **dissonance** or psychological discomfort for the individual
- *Naive scientist*: This is where people try to understand other people by generating inferences or hypotheses like scientists. It is the area within which the attribution theories developed
- *Cognitive misers*: This model developed in response to the naive scientist as it was found people had limited processing capacity and so developed shortcuts to understanding others by using **heuristics** or 'rules of thumb'
- *Motivated tactician*: This model developed from the cognitive miser model and in response to the consistency model. It acknowledges the role of emotion and motivation in perception

Cognitive social perception also involves a group of theories that have been called 'attribution theories'.

Attribution theories

The correspondent theory

Attribution theories accept the person as a naive scientist, and that they are logical, rational, thinking beings. It is important to recognise that this is not the assumption made by all psychological perspectives; for example think about the psychodynamic theory. Jones and Davis (1965) developed an attribution theory called the 'correspondent theory'. They indicate that people make **correspondent inferences**. This is where an observed behaviour closely relates to an identified personality trait – they correspond. Inferences about people's behaviour are based on the disposition of the person (their personality/traits) and intentionality (that behaviour exhibited gained the intended response). The disposition of the person is assessed by the distinction between one choice of behaviour and another.

Influences on the assessment of disposition are:

- Choice
- Social desirability
- Roles
- Prior expectations

✺ Ali

Ali is a 25-year-old occupational therapist who is new in post. His parents were also involved in healthcare as his father was a GP and his mother is a physiotherapist, and Ali always wanted to work in the caring profession. Ali currently works in a neurological ward in a large general hospital. He has become increasingly concerned about the behaviour of one of his clients, Fred, who was a very active 64-year-old prior to admission. Fred is extremely frustrated by his condition, which has greatly impacted on his capacity to undertake his preferred occupations. This has been expressed in frequent verbally aggressive outbursts on the ward to staff and visitors. Ali has found Fred to be very uncooperative and negative when Ali attempts to assess Fred in his self-care activities.

This behaviour has left Ali feeling frustrated and incompetent and the idealism which accompanied him to his first post is rapidly ebbing. He feels inadequate but is reluctant to discuss this with his clinical supervisor as he feels that it will reflect poorly on him. He is feeling increasingly vulnerable and isolated and is reluctant to re-engage with Fred.

If we consider the behaviour of Fred in the case study of Ali, we can assume that Fred has some choice in his behaviour and certainly Ali appears to believe this. His behaviour is not socially desirable and does not correspond to the expectations that Ali had of the patients he would work with. This situation could have led Ali to believe that Fred was a difficult person and that his behaviour is due to his personality (attribute behaviour to disposition), whereas Ali appears to attribute Fred's behaviour to his current condition – given his assumed behaviour prior to admission and the behaviour not achieving what Ali believes Fred is trying to achieve (intentionality). Ali believes that he should be able to care for Fred, given this belief.

Kelley's covariance models

Kelley's (1967) covariance model refers to the dispositional characteristics a person is seen to have when something is known of the person and of the social norms for the particular behaviour. The decisions made about dispositions are based on:

- *Consensus*: Would other people behave in the same way? If so, then the behaviour is seen as a social norm
- *Distinctiveness*: Is this something that the person only does in certain circumstances? If so, then this is seen as a situational response
- *Consistency*: How often does the person exhibit this behaviour? If it is something which they frequently do, it can be seen as a dispositional characteristic

Kelley suggests that when consensus is low, distinctiveness is low, but consistency is high, the casual attribution will be to the actor, in this case the care practitioner. In other words, if the behaviour is something that is consistently done just by this care practitioner, then it is attributed to their disposition. If it is something that is done by lots of people (consensus high) in this situation (distinctiveness high) and only in this situation (consistency low), then circumstances would be the casual attribution or a situational reason.

So, if we return to the case study of Ali and re-examine Fred and Ali's behaviour, we can see that Fred's behaviour is low on consensus (other people are not behaving like this on this ward), distinctiveness is low (he is exhibiting this behaviour in a variety of situations) and consistency is high (Fred is exhibiting this behaviour most of the time). This would lead people to believe that Fred's behaviour is something to do with his disposition, and may lead the caregiver to respond in an uncaring manner, like in this case study avoiding care provision.

Ali's concerns about his supervisor's understanding of his behaviour can also be explored using this theory. Are the other care practitioners also avoiding Fred? Is this something that Ali does just in this situation? How often does Ali avoid care provision? If Ali observes others providing care for Fred and that Fred is less aggressive with them, this could lead Ali to attribute to his disposition his inability to offer care and believe his supervisor will do the same thing.

Activity 6.5   Critical thinking

If you were in Ali's position, how might you behave towards Fred?

An outline answer is available at the end of the chapter.

Whilst this theory makes logical and rationale sense we need to be aware that even the theorists advocating this theory have noticed that people have biases.

Fundamental attribution error

This is sometimes known as the 'correspondence bias' or 'attribution effect'. This occurs when we make judgements or attribution about other people's behaviour or our own behaviour. We exhibit an error or bias in these attributions: when we consider the reason for our own behaviour we usually attribute it to external factors, whereas when we consider other people's behaviour we usually attribute them to internal factors.

If we return to Ali's case study, we find that Ali is attributing Fred's aggressive behaviour to his health problems and so to an internal cause, whereas he is attributing his avoidance of Fred to Fred's behaviour. Likewise, if we return to the case study of Mel, we can see that Chris appears to attribute Mel's behaviour to a lack of skills or motivation, whereas he attributes his behaviour or lack of engagement to Mel's reluctance.

This bias can be seen to be explained through a lack of knowledge of the person and the situation. For Chris and Ali they can reflect on what is happening to themselves and identify detailed external factors which they are also focusing on in the situation. However, they may have a little knowledge of all the factors influencing Mel's and Fred's behaviour and their focus is on Mel and Fred, rather than on everything that is going on around them.

How are others perceived?

Attribution theory offers one explanation of how others are seen. It explains how inferences are made about people's behaviour leading to perception of dispositional characteristics through certain rules, but there are alternative theories of how others are perceived.

Implicit personality theories can be used or clusters of traits. These can offer shortcuts when there is little information available to make an accurate assessment; some of these methods are:

- Halo effect
- Stereotyping
- Importance of names
- Importance of physical appearance

Solomon Asch in the 1940s and 1950s conducted extensive research into conformity. In an experiment in 1946 he demonstrated the importance of two key dispositional characteristics – warm and cold. He called this the **halo effect**. If someone was labelled 'warm', then a number of other characteristics would be attributed to them – the positive halo. If someone had been labelled 'cold' regardless of other characteristics, then they gained a negative halo and this led to other negative characteristics being attributed to them.

Names and physical appearance also generate consistent groups of characteristics but appear to be culturally sensitive. For example, 30 years ago, if a person was fat they were considered jolly, but when children are asked what a fat person is like in the twenty-first century, the children would see this person as selfish and greedy. Certain names are also associated with certain personality types; for example Matthew is seen in a more positive light than Wayne.

These could be considered stereotypes but usually this term is reserved for whole social groups rather than individuals. There is disagreement about the usefulness of stereotypes as they can lead to discrimination. They can also be used as mental shortcuts within normal cognitive functioning.

How do we influence how others perceive us?

In order to engage and maintain the trust of those they are caring for, all care practitioners need to demonstrate a professional manner. Therefore, it is important that care practitioners are aware of how they can influence other people's perceptions of themselves. Alongside unconscious attributions, social perceptions are influenced in a number of ways:

- Impression management
- Self-presentation
- Consistency
- Self-monitoring
- Self-disclosure

Impression management and self-presentation involve a certain level of emotional intelligence (see Chapter 8) as the necessary techniques used need self-awareness and understanding others' feelings or perceptions, which can be termed 'empathy' (see Chapter 7). Once this is achieved, they need to **self-regulate** using their **social skills**. Techniques used to achieve impression management include **behaviour matching**, appreciating and complimenting others. Demonstrating internal consistency is also important.

Self-monitors are in a continuous cycle of assessing and managing themselves. As with impression management, they use their self-awareness, empathy and social skills to self-regulate by coming alongside others and 'being' what others need and expect of them. Low self-monitors or self-regulators could be considered lacking in social skills but they could be considered to have greater personal integrity as they are consistent in their behaviour, not adjusting these to make a good impression.

Self-disclosure partly determines how other people see us, and there has been debate within services about whether care practitioners should disclose information about themselves. The usual rules influencing self-disclosure in personal relationships – such as reciprocity, trust, quality of the relationship and gender, influencing self-disclosure within families and friendships – may not apply to professional relationships.

Self-disclosure is seen as a significant area where boundaries are broken or violated but there are clear guidelines available despite the limited research in the area; for example Baca (2011) identifies that disclosure should not be used:

- If it discloses the caregiver's current needs or problems
- If disclosure occurs regularly
- When there is no clear connection to the problems or experiences with which the caregiver is dealing
- When it is not likely to provide encouragement or support
- If it comprises more than a few minutes of the person's time
- If it occurs despite apparent confusion for the listener

Despite this, within certain care environments, self-disclosure is becoming more acceptable, for example in care of people with dementia and midwifery: Rogers' call for congruence in caregivers (Barker, 2007), Hunter's (2006) recognition of the usefulness of reciprocal relationships in midwifery care, and the call for being open and real in relationships with people with dementia (Barker and Board, 2012).

Summary

This section has considered the psychological theories related to perception. Key elements of social perception, particularly attribution of behaviour to personality or situation, helps care practitioners reflect on their own behaviour as well as that of others. The use of stereotypes, self-presentation, self-monitoring and self-disclosure was also considered in relation to care practitioners. In the next section, attitudes are explored because it is believed that there is a link between attitudes and behaviours, including showing care.

Attitudes

Allport (1935) described 'attitudes' as the single most important concept in social psychology and offered the following definition of it as: 'a mental or neural state of readiness, organised through experience, exerting a directive or dynamic influence upon the individual's response to all objects and situations with which it is related' (Allport, 1935: 810). This definition falls within a cognitive empirical approach. If, as Allport states, attitudes influence people's behaviour, then its relevance in the study of health and social care cannot be overestimated. It is not generally agreed or established in research, however, that attitudes do influence or predict behaviour. Some theorists suggest that behaviour influences attitudes (Hogg and Vaughan, 2005).

Attitudes, beliefs and values are all closely related, so they will be differentiated before attitudes are explored in more depth:

- *Attitude*: An attitude is an evaluation of something – which may be a person or an object, abstract or concrete – which prepares the individual to respond to it. Attitudes normally have a value placed on them which can be negative or positive
- *Beliefs*: A belief is something we hold to be true about the world. Beliefs can be abstract and allied to another belief or within a cluster, for example within a religious system. Beliefs are also understood in terms of opinion and acceptance as they cannot always be supported by scientific evidence but are supported by **faith**.
- *Values*: Strongly related to beliefs, and affecting attitudes, values are linked to the moral or ethical standards a person lives by

Components of attitudes

There is some discussion between social psychologists about the number of components of attitudes, but there is a general acceptance that they include:

- Affective – emotion
- Cognitive – thought
- Behaviour – past experiences of attitudinal object

There is an interrelationship between attitudes, values and beliefs and all are very difficult to alter. Attitudes could be considered the emotional, cognitive or behavioural response to beliefs influenced by the values of the person (Barker, 2007).

Functions of attitude

Attitudes can be useful for the person in three ways as they:

- Allow the person to make sense of the world
- Offer a heuristic or simple strategy for understanding an object
- Provide a structure to guide the memory

Attitudes influence people's thoughts, feelings and behaviours in many areas such as lifestyle choices, consumer activity, voting and political behaviour, and even interpersonal attraction. Given this theoretical understanding, the impact of attitudes on those providing care and those receiving care could be significant and could precipitate:

- Fear of hospitals, doctors, nurses or various medical treatments
- Awe of doctors and nurses, which may lead to submissive behaviour and reduced self-efficacy
- A negative response to health information such as smoking cessation and safe sex
- Prejudice towards certain groups of people such as people who self-harm or who are obese or have a learning disability

There have been numerous studies exploring attitudes to a wide variety of care issues, as there continues to be an expected link between attitudes and behaviour. If attitudes are considered a heuristic or shortcut, it may be short-sighted to organise care around them. Attitudes are usually explored using empirical statistical research methods and, whilst giving a broad overview, they do not help care practitioners understand or support people as unique individuals. To understand a person's thoughts, feelings and beliefs, care practitioners need to develop a relationship in which they carefully listen to the person's story as indicated by person-centred approaches.

Summary

This section has considered what constitutes an attitude, how it is formed and what function it may perform. It was acknowledged that cognitive psychologists indicate that there is an interrelationship between attitudes, values and beliefs. Whilst the section concluded that attitudes could be considered a useful starting point in the understanding of people and their behaviour, it would be ineffective in consider the care needs of individuals.

Stereotyping and prejudice

As highlighted above, attitudes are not all neutral or benign; people can hold both positive and negative attitudes: thought, feelings or beliefs about objects and others. Whilst positive attitudes are said to be enhancing to well-being, negative attitudes can lead to prejudice and discrimination.

Stereotyping is defined as a widely shared simple evaluation of a social group. It attributes certain characteristics to that social group. Stereotypes usually have the following shared attributes:

- They are applied to an easily identified group due to for example skin colour, where a person lives or their ability
- It is believed that all members of this group share certain characteristics
- It is believed that a particular individual has these characteristics

There has been debate about whether stereotyping is useful or problematic. It was suggested that placing individuals in stereotyped groups did not allow for the recognition of individuality as no two people in a group are exactly the same: the cultural hegemony enforces every person as unique. It has also been recognised that stereotyping can facilitate rapid evaluation or judgements and reduces the toll on limited cognitive capacity. The movement towards person-centred care and self-management of long-term conditions, however, should discourage care practitioners from using this strategy in their care practices.

Care practitioners frequently need to deal with issues of stigmatism and prejudice occurring towards the people with whom they work. **Stigma** refers to a person with a visible sign that they belong to a certain group or are outside of the dominant group. There are many groups within society who experience prejudice and discrimination, including:

- Certain racial or religious groups
- People who have certain physical deformities, diseases or amputations

- People who experience mental illness or disability
- People of differing sexual orientations
- Certain occupations

Care practitioners are expected to work with all racial and religious groups and all occupations and sexual orientations so they will need to consider issues of discrimination that may be expressed towards the people they are caring for. They also need to self-monitor so as to assess whether their behaviour is being affected by any negative stereotypes which they themselves hold.

Care practitioners also need to work with people to reduce their self-stigma, as identified by Rogers many people who are unwell despise themselves, holding self-stigmas. Self-stigmas involve stereotypes, prejudice and discrimination:

- *Stereotype*: Negative beliefs about the self, such as character weakness, incompetence
- *Prejudice*: Response to negative belief, negative emotional reaction, such as low self-esteem, low self-efficacy
- *Discrimination*: Behavioural response to prejudice, such as failing to pursue work and housing opportunities (Corrigan and Watson, 2002)

Care practitioners need to be aware of not only their own stereotypes and prejudices that may lead to stigma but also of those of the people they are caring for so that they can facilitate the person's self-worth and self-esteem. This can be achieved through person-centred compassionate care (see Chapter 4).

Chapter summary

This chapter explored the character of the care practitioner through psychological theory and research. This was achieved through identifying and describing personality theories from the psychodynamic, behavioural, cognitive and humanistic perspectives. Self-concept was discussed along with the associated concepts of self-esteem and self-awareness. It was identified that self-awareness and self-esteem were necessary for care practitioners to provide person-centred compassionate care.

Motivation related to becoming and remaining well was explored for each of the psychological perspectives, leading to an examination of perception. Most of the perceptual theories were from the cognitive perspective, which offers limited understanding of the individual.

Attribution theories for interpreting behaviour can help the caregiver but are limited in the provision of compassionate care. Finally, the chapter considered attitudes, stereotyping and stigma. Whilst attitude theories are again mostly cognitive, these did lead to considering the impact of stereotyping, prejudice and stigma, which are important issues that can be addressed through person-centred compassionate care.

Further study

The Social Care Institute of Excellence (SCIE) website offers a valuable resource: it provides television clips, e-learning packages and policy guidance, and also sponsors research into care. Their aim is to facilitate the opportunity for inclusiveness for all who live within the community. They work collaboratively with people receiving care to ensure provision fulfils their needs. They provide guidance to safeguard individuals from stigma and discrimination by supporting their self-efficacy, self-esteem and self-worth. See: www.scie.org.uk/about/

Activity outline answers

Activity 6.1   Critical thinking

When you were young, did your family say that they could see you becoming a firefighter, farmer, doctor, nanny? If they did, why did they suggest this?

It is likely, if your family identified that you would be good at caring for people, that they described your behaviour using words like:

- Kind, helpful, practical

And your disposition such as:

- Patient, understanding, sensible, good

Whilst many of these stereotypes of people in caring professions still exist, there have been more negative stereotypes recently.

Likewise for farmers, you may have enjoyed the company of animals, and firefighters are usually seen as protective and brave.

Activity 6.2   Critical thinking

- How would you describe your personality?
- Do you describe it in terms of feeling? Likes, dislikes?
- Do you describe it in terms of abilities?
- Do you describe it in terms of what you do?
- Who am I and what gives meaning to my life?

You could have used any of the above and they would give you insight into your values and priorities in life.

People usually describe their personality by identifying internal dispositions such as:

- Kind, caring, inquisitive, understanding, resilient, motivated

Activity 6.5   Critical thinking

If you were in Ali's position, how might you behave towards Fred?

It is clear that Fred is frustrated with his situation: this will be causing him a great deal of stress, leading to his agitated and aggressive behaviour. A person-centred approach would encourage you to spend some time with Fred to develop understanding of him, and to find out what makes him most frustrated and what makes him feel calmer. Once you have engaged with him by taking his frustrations and feelings seriously, you may be able to start undertaking some basic problem-solving. It may be with some imagination that Fred can be supported to undertake some of the activities he enjoys.

References

Allport, G.W. (1935) 'Attitudes', in C.A. Murchison (ed.), *A Handbook of Social Psychology*. New York: Russell & Russell, pp. 789–844.

Asch, S.E. (1946) 'Forming impressions of personality', *Journal of Abnormal and Social Psychology*, 41: 258–90.

Baca, M. (2011) 'Professional boundaries and dual relationships in clinical practice', *Journal for Nurse Practitioners*, 7 (3): 195–200.

Bandura, A. (1965) 'Influence of model's reinforcement contingencies on the acquisition of imitative responses', *Journal of Personality & Psychology*, 1: 589–95.

Barker, S. (2007) *Vital Notes for Nurses: Psychology*. Oxford: Blackwell.

Barker, S. and Board, M. (2012) *Dementia Care in Nursing*. Exeter: Learning Matters.

Corrigan, P.W. and Watson, A.C. (2002) 'Understanding the impact of stigma on people with mental illness', *World Psychiatry*, 1 (1): 16–20.

Gibson, J.J. (1966) *The Senses Considered as Perceptual Systems*. Boston, MA: Houghton.

Goffman, I. (1971) *The Presentation of Self in Everyday Life*. Harmondsworth: Penguin.

Gregory, R.L. (1966) *Eye and Brain*. London: Weidenfeld & Nicholson.

Hogg, M. and Vaughan, G. (2005) *Social Psychology*, 3rd edn. London: Prentice Hall.

Hunter, B. (2006) 'The importance of reciprocity in relationships between community-based midwives and mothers', *Midwifery*, 22 (4): 308–22. Available at: www.sciencedirect.com (accessed September 2015).

Jones, E.E. and Davis, K.E. (1965) 'From acts to dispositions: The attribution process in person perception', in L. Berkowitz (ed.), *Advances in Experimental Social Psychology*, Vol. 2. New York: Academic Press, pp. 219–66.

Kelley, H.H. (1967) 'Attribution theory in social psychology', in D. Levine (ed.), *Nebraska Symposium on Motivation*. Lincoln, NB: University of Nebraska Press, pp. 192–238.

Maslow, A. (1954) *Motivation and Personality*. New York: Harper and Row.

Neisser, U. (1976) *Cognition and Reality*. San Franscico, CA: W.H. Freeman.

Rogers, C.R. (1951) *Client-Centred Therapy*. London: Constable.

Rogers, C.R. (1961) *A Therapist's View of Psychotherapy: On Becoming a Person*. London: Constable.

Stewart, W. (2005) *An A–Z of Counselling Theory and Practice*. Cheltenham: Nelson Thornes.

7 Therapeutic Relationships

Sue Barker and Hamed Al Battashi

I was stumbling in the dark
Pain and sadness in my heart
Your listening felt warm and safe
Your gentle compassion at my pace
Opened my eyes to a world of what I could be
For the first time, I saw Me!

Learning objectives

All care practitioners need to engage in relationships with those for whom they care. This relationship is usually considered a helping relationship and therefore therapeutic. Given the essentially therapeutic nature of these relationships, it is important that care practitioners have an understanding of how to manage these to enhance their helping. This chapter's learning objectives are to:

- Discuss the differing explanations and interventions for each of the psychological perspectives underpinning therapeutic relationships
- Identify why self-awareness is important within the therapeutic relationship
- Recognise the core elements of a therapeutic relationship

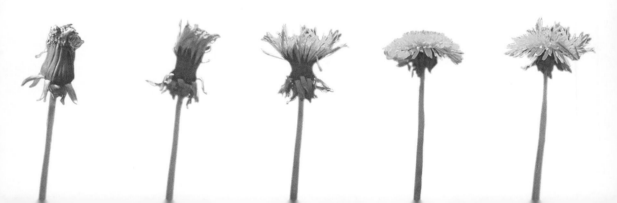

Introduction

The focus of this chapter is how and why care practitioners might develop and utilise therapeutic relationships. It will consider each of the psychological perspectives and explore the understanding they can provide. It will explain the core components of any therapeutic relationship, highlighting the relationship between these and their psychological underpinning. Case studies will be used to enhance understanding of how psychological knowledge can be applied within care practices.

Whilst the chapter explores each psychological perspective's associated therapeutic approaches, this does not mean that they are equally valid: some 'therapies' may be considered unethical using a life world, person-centred approach.

Activity 7.1   Reflection

Take a few minutes to think about your caring role:

- How would you define it?
- Would you say that 'counselling' was part of your role?
- Would you say that you developed therapeutic relationships with the people for whom you are providing care?

As this is a reflection, there is no outline answer at the end of the chapter.

The term **therapeutic relationship** is used extensively in care, but what counts as a therapeutic relationship? Is this a **counselling** relationship or is it something more basic such as any helping endeavours that are negotiated between two people, like collecting a person's shopping? The terms 'therapeutic', 'counselling' and 'helping relationship' at times appear to be used interchangeably.

If a dictionary or thesaurus is used to examine each of these terms, 'therapeutic' is acknowledged as something to do with treatment, which may involve counselling. It can also include activities such as giving advice, medication or meals; it involves enabling or assisting. In fact, care practitioners could be seen to be supporting all activities of daily living, including those related to physical or psychological care.

Psychological theorists refer to the terms 'therapeutic relationship', the 'counselling relationship' and the 'helping relationship', not in the eclectic manner used by many healthcare practitioners, but more specifically, giving each type of relationship some distinction. This leads to different care professions or disciplines adopting one or other of these titles (Barker, 2007).

This chapter will primarily use the term 'therapeutic relationship', with the understanding that 'therapeutic' is to do with offering appropriate treatment, whether that is offering advice, administering medication or aiding activities of daily living. This will be explored through the relationship that care practitioners engage in. This book acknowledges that each care practitioner relationship is unique but they can all be supported or informed by psychological theory.

Each of the psychological perspectives offer a different approach to managing the therapeutic relationship but one thing that all approaches expect is that the person managing the relationship has some awareness of themselves: self-awareness.

Self-awareness is being conscious of one's own existence or life world. It is about being able to accurately perceive one's own physical body, thoughts, feelings, spirituality and actions within their embodied time and space.

Self-awareness

The development of self-awareness is a choice, but once the choice has been made it has consequences for the care practitioner, although some would suggest that, to be caring, self-awareness is essential. Once the development of self-understanding is started, the practitioner may need to address issues about themselves that were not, originally, in their consciousness.

Self-awareness can be achieved through techniques such as reflective practice. Care practitioners can be taught models of reflection to guide them but most registered or chartered practitioners are expected to continue to develop these skills. **Reflection** can also be used as part of clinical supervision (see Chapter 10).

There are numerous elements that influence an individual's behaviour and it may be useful to reflect on these to develop self-awareness. These include:

- Thoughts
- Feelings
- Behaviour
- Beliefs
- Attitudes
- Values
- Hopes and fears
- Likes and dislikes
- Past experiences

Activity 7.2　Reflection

Explore how you think, feel and respond (behave) related to your beliefs, attitudes, values, hopes, fears, likes, dislikes and past experiences of your caring role.

As this is a reflection, there is no outline answer at the end of the chapter.

Developing self-awareness can be seen as a lifelong undertaking and those with greater awareness could be considered to be more mature, but chronological age does not necessarily correlate to self-awareness (see Chapter 6).

Luft and Ingham (1955) developed a model which suggests four quadrants of awareness; It is called the 'Johari window' (see Figure 7.1). This model indicates that there are parts of ourselves that are kept private, and parts that can only be seen by

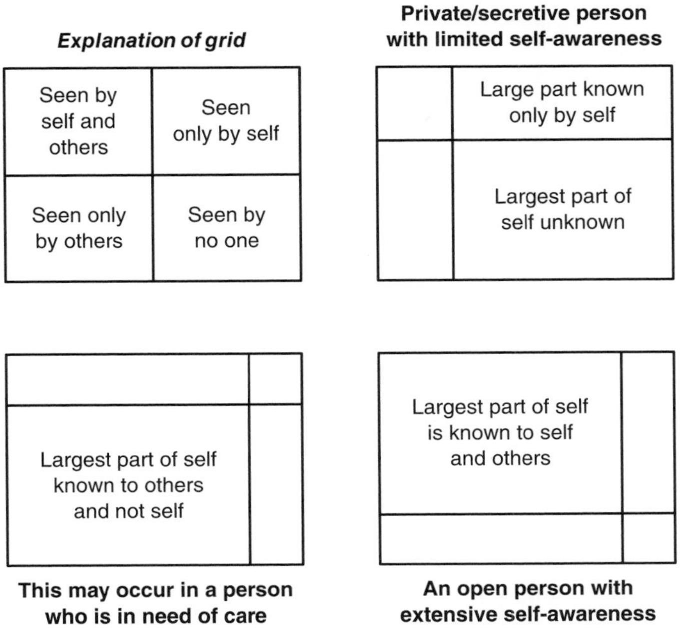

Explanation of grid

Seen by self and others	Seen only by self
Seen only by others	Seen by no one

Private/secretive person with limited self-awareness

	Large part known only by self
	Largest part of self unknown

Largest part of self known to others and not self	

This may occur in a person who is in need of care

Largest part of self is known to self and others	

An open person with extensive self-awareness

Figure 7.1   A simplified version of the Johari window

others, but also that there is a part of the self that cannot be seen by ourselves or others. This might be considered the unconscious part of the self, but only some psychological theorists accept the concept of the unconscious mind and that the self is not totally open to the person. In therapy or therapeutic relationships, the aim is to enable the person to be aware of their understanding of themselves and make changes to it if they find that it would facilitate their well-being.

Psychodynamic approaches to managing the therapeutic relationship

The development of self-awareness can be traced back to the work of Freud, who was particularly concerned with unconscious processes and how they influenced the experience of the present. His psychoanalytic approach to therapy involved bringing to consciousness the experiences that had been repressed so that they could be addressed and the person could continue to grow – increasing their self-awareness.

Freud outlined that behaviours are guided by the three conflicting components of the mind or psyche (see Chapters 1 and 2): the id, ego and superego. He suggested that the unconscious drives of the id are the motivating forces in a person's life. These he called the 'life drives' (Eros) and 'death drives' (Thanos). The motivating force for the life drive is 'libido': Freud believed that this motivation for sexual fulfilment was present at birth.

Care practitioners – as with other people at times – use mental defence mechanisms to deal with these drives within their social environment to manage the inner conflict caused by not fulfilling these needs immediately (see Chapter 1). Mental defence mechanisms can resolve the unfulfilled need in the short term, but in the longer term the need must be addressed.

Psychoanalysis suggests that needs and desires unmet in childhood will affect the adult personality, and to resolve problems in the adult personality these unconscious needs or desires should be brought to conscious awareness. There are four techniques that are used to achieve this:

- Free association
- Dream analysis
- Transference
- Information leakage such as parapraxes (also known as 'Freudian slips') (Barker, 2007)

The psychoanalyst uses this information to interpret the problems for the person. Their interpretation is then given to the client to enable them to manage their lives. Whilst care practitioners may not in general use psychoanalysis (it takes many years to train to become a psychoanalyst) in managing their therapeutic relationships with clients, there are some techniques that psychoanalysis offers which might be useful.

Transference

This is where a client transfers onto the analyst their feelings and sometimes consequential behaviours about a significant person in their lives. The analyst may in turn through countertransference respond to the client as if they were a significant person in the analyst's life such as their daughter, mother, etc. The analyst can use this information to understand and interpret the person's problems. This can be a useful tool but it can occur in other therapeutic relationships that are not intended to be psychodynamic; they are non-analytic situations and create confusion and frustration for client and care practitioner. If care practitioners are aware that transference and countertransference might occur in their therapeutic relationships, it may allow them to manage these more effectively.

Countertransference

Transference refers to when clients project their thoughts, feelings and behaviours onto the therapist but countertransference can also occur. This is where the therapist projects their thoughts, feeling or behaviours towards the client. This may occur in response to the client triggering early traumas for the therapist or because of the therapist's current needs. To reduce the risk of countertransference, care practitioners are usually encouraged professionally not to disclose personal information.

Summary

Although most care practitioners will not use a psychodynamic approach to therapy with the people they are caring for, it can offer understanding for them about themselves and others. This approach to therapeutic relationships is not an even one, as the power is with the therapist who is the expert and interprets what the client is saying. Whilst individual, it is not in essence person-centred compassionate care. This approach does not accept the therapist sharing personal information due to the risk of transference and countertransference. Person-centred compassionate care does accept the usefulness of self-disclosure but it is helpful if care practitioners are mindful of countertransference.

Behavioural approaches to managing the therapeutic relationship

The behavioural psychologists believe that babies are born with the in-built ability to learn and that all their behaviour, including language, is learned (see Chapters 1 and 2). The behaviourists particularly focus on the relationship between the person or animal and their environment. Most of their research was conducted with animals. This learning occurs at a primitive level by habituation through to classical conditioning and then operant conditioning to social learning theory. Each of these stages can be seen as hierarchical:

1. Habituation is learning by familiarisation
2. Classical conditioning is learning by repetition and pairing (association and law of exercise)
3. Operant conditioning is learning through reinforcement and punishment (reward)
4. Social learning theory is learning by observation and imitation (vicarious)

Classical conditioning

This was established by Pavlov (1927), where conditioning or learning occurs when a person reflexively responds to a given stimulus. The reflexive response can be trained (conditioned) to occur with a previously unassociated stimulus by repeated pairing with it. Hence this can be referred to as 'learning by association': if one stimulus is associated with another stimulus that produces a certain response, after a period of time, both stimuli will gain the same response. For example, painkillers are given at the same time as an **inert substance** such as a sugar tablet. The two stimuli are associated and after a while the painkiller can be removed but the person still experiences the pain relief. Both painkiller and sugar tablet have the same response. This is classical conditioning or learning by association.

Operant conditioning

Thorndike (1913) developed the concept of instrumental conditioning, accepting the principles of Pavlov but introducing the element of reinforcement. This development was continued by Skinner (1938) and became operant conditioning. This approach is based on the **law of effect**, which states that when something good happens after an action the behaviour is likely to be repeated. The characteristics of classical conditioning still occur but behavioural shaping through **successive approximation** is also said to occur in operant conditioning. Learning occurs when a person is rewarded. If they are rewarded for behaviour, then they will re-enact the behaviour and are said to have learned that behaviour. This can be seen in many animals as well as people. Skinner suggested that in the real world, animals do not just respond to one stimulus and so he looked at how they operated within their environments. Both of these theories of learning can assist the care practitioner in their understanding their therapeutic relationships.

In operant conditioning, learning is either achieved through training by a teacher or as a matter of 'trial and error'; in either situation rewards or punishment influence the learning and future behaviour. There have been a number of therapies in care services that have developed from these two learning theories as well as strategies in education.

Therapies based on classical conditioning are:

- **Systematic desensitisation**
- Aversion therapy
- Exposure therapy

Therapies based on operant conditioning are:

- Behaviour modification
- Token economies
- Stimulus satiation

Systematic desensitisation (classical conditioning)

This approach can be used with objects or situations that provoke fear or anxiety. The assumption is that the person's fear or anxiety is based on maladaptive learning or unhelpful associations and so the person needs to relearn or form new associations. 'Systematic' refers to a graded introduction to the feared situation and 'desensitisation' refers to the **counterbalancing** or reducing of the fear response. Counterbalancing can be achieved by activities such as **progressive relaxation** or medication. An example could be being introduced gradually to spiders to overcome a fear of them.

Aversion therapy (classical conditioning)

This therapeutic approach is used to extinguish unwanted behaviours such as alcohol abuse or sexual deviance. Many techniques have been used to create an unpleasant response (punishment) when doing the undesired behaviour. For a person abusing alcohol, medication such an Antabuse (disulfiram) can be prescribed which induces a feeling of being very unwell: they become hot with flushing, feel nauseous and vomit when they drink alcohol. Elastic bands have been used; they are worn around the wrist and the person 'pings' themselves with it if they do something they should not. These are to develop negative associations for the behaviour to be extinguished. Whilst this 'therapy' offers a commonsense approach, care practitioners are frequently uncomfortable with engaging in an activity that might cause harm, because we subscribe the biomedical ethic of non-maleficence. There is also limited evidence to support the efficacy of punishments producing long-term behavioural changes.

Exposure therapy (classical conditioning)

This is where the feared stimulus (object or situation) is repeatedly presented to the person without giving them the opportunity to respond and so the fear response/behaviour becomes **extinct**.

Behavioural modification (operant conditioning)

As this therapeutic approach is derived from operant conditioning, the focus is to reinforce desired behaviours. A behavioural plan can be drawn up with specific goals. Once the baseline behaviours are established, the behavioural strategy identified in the plan can be put into action. The plan needs to have small sub-goals on the path towards the overall goals. Each sub-goal is reinforced (rewarded) until it is an established behaviour to slowly shape behaviour towards the main behavioural goal.

Token economies (operant conditioning)

Again, this uses the approach of reinforcing desired behaviours. In this case, a token is used to reinforce the behaviour. Most schools use this approach with the children (star charts and house points) and it has been used in psychiatric hospitals (tokens which can be redeemed at the hospital shop). It can also be seen in the use of loyalty cards in supermarkets and in modular degree programmes – collecting marks to gain an average that will lead to a good honours classification.

Stimulus satiation (operant conditioning)

This therapeutic approach again uses the concept of reinforcement and punishment, as with all operant conditioning. For this approach, though, they are used in a counter-intuitive way. Instead of punishing the problematic behaviour to ameliorate it, it is rewarded. The reinforcement is over-used, as too much of anything can become a reason for extinguishing behaviour (Figure 7.2). The desire is satiated and so the behaviour stops; it is extinct.

Social learning theory

Another form of learning that builds on classical and operant conditioning is social learning theory, which acknowledged a cognitive element to learning (see Chapter 1). The theory suggests that learning can occur not only by association and reward but also by observing others' behaviour and imitating it – vicarious learning.

Albert Bandura (1977) and colleagues developed the theory of social learning through a number of experiments. These demonstrated that observational or vicarious learning could occur. For this type of learning to take place, there needs to be another person or people to learn from this person, who is usually referred to as the 'role model'.

Role-modelling can be important as part of the therapeutic relationship. If the care practitioner wishes to influence a person's behaviour through their therapeutic relationships, then they could become a role model.

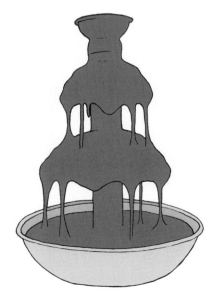

Figure 7.2 Is this enough chocolate?

Activity 7.3 Critical thinking

Think about a person whom you admired and wanted to be like. What did they do, how did they make you feel and what responses did they get?

See the case study of Alison as an example of this.

Case study

 Alison

As a foster carer, I was visiting a foster home of a foster mother who is no longer able to care for the little boy who was staying with her due to her health problems. Social services had identified me and my husband as appropriate alternative carers. The social worker and I arrived and the little boy was fearful and trying to hide behind the foster mother. I felt very concerned for him. The social worker tried to engage with him but he would not talk to her. We chatted (the foster mother, social worker and I) for a little time. The foster mother asked me some questions that seemed a little odd but I answered her honestly. After a short while, she said to the little boy, 'Did you know that Alison's husband has the same name as you and he has a quad bike!' The little boy's face brightened and he asked me what colour it was, whilst still holding her hand. I had my phone with me that had some photos of my husband with the quad bike and some of our animals. The boy gradually started asking about the animals and moved on to where he would sleep and what food he likes, and occasionally looked at the foster mother for reassurance.

Effective role models

There are certain features that make a role model effective. These features enhance the vicarious learning. An effective role model has the following attributes:

- *They are rewarded*: Alison could see that the little boy trusted the foster mother
- *They are similar enough to imitate*: Alison felt she could imitate the foster mother's patience and attention to finding out what would help the little boy feel better about what was happening
- *They have a positive status*: Foster mothers are generally portrayed positively, and for Alison it was a role she wanted to take on; so for her, foster mothers had a positive status

This would suggest that for a carer to be a good role model and to develop a therapeutic relationship, they need to be similar to the people they are working with, to be liked and appear to be rewarded. Bandura (1977) also identified that, along with the concrete skills or behaviours which can be learned using this approach, people can develop their values and attitudes, along with problem-solving and self-evaluation.

Almahdi Hussain

Almahdi was admitted to the drug addiction unit for heroin abuse detoxification. The treatment plan was to provide buprenorphine. Almahdi reported insomnia to the treating team but the doctor refused to prescribe any night sedation to help him sleep. Whilst this might be a side effect of the medication the psychiatrist rationalised his decision to the team by saying that Almahdi was probably lying and trying to manipulate them to get more sedation. The psychiatrist expressed the belief that drug addicts are not trustworthy, and that they are demanding, dishonest and manipulative people. The team appeared to accept this explanation and ignored Almahdi's requests.

Almahdi became angry, shouting at the team that they did not understand him or his problems. He then signed his own discharge against medical advice. It was obvious that he was frustrated and agitated when he left the unit. Later that day, Almahdi was found in his room at home unconscious and bleeding from both his arms. He was successfully treated at the local hospital and then returned to the addiction unit. The team was surprised to hear about his reaction after being discharged from the unit. The team believed that this was a serious attempt at ending his life and so when he returned they put effort into developing a therapeutic relationship with him to understand how to help him.

Consider the case study of Almahdi Hussain. It can be seen that the psychiatrist was an influential role model for the team. Even if the team did not share his beliefs about people with addiction problems, they behaved in a way that indicated to Almahdi that they did. The team could have continued to accept the negative attitudes of the psychiatrist but when they saw the harm to Almahdi the psychiatrist's values and attitudes could be considered not to be rewarded and at that point their status would also have been less positive.

Self-efficacy

Self-efficacy is an important factor in prompting a behaviour or motivation. For social learning or vicarious learning to be effective, a person's motivation to attempt imitation is dependent on their belief that they can achieve the behaviour: self-efficacy. Self-efficacy is usually developed from previous experiences of the same or similar situations. It is important that care practitioners are aware of and develop not only their own self-efficacy to motivate their caregiving, but also that of the people with whom they work to achieve positive outcomes. If we return to the case study of Almahdi, he did not appear to believe that he could achieve withdrawal from heroin without the additional support. This can be seen to lead to his no longer attempting to stay at the unit and undertake the withdrawal process and his inability to manage at home. It may also be that, given previous experiences, the psychiatrist and team did not feel that they were going to be successful in the treatment of Almahdi as he was already asking for more medication.

Summary

Behavioural approaches to therapy offer the student care practitioner an insight into what influences people's behaviour, including their own. Classical conditioning demonstrates the importance of staying in a fearful situation until the fear has been extinguished, and that responses to stimuli will determine whether behaviour continues: stimulus–response theory. Operant conditioning highlights the importance of reinforcement (especially positive reinforcement or reward) to facilitate continuation of behaviour. Social learning theory highlights the efficacy of vicarious learning, the use of role models and self-efficacy.

Most behavioural therapists are highly skilled individuals with extensive training, although many of these techniques are used by people in everyday life. It is important to recognise, though, that the relationship between therapist and client is not even because the therapist has the power and manipulates the person's behaviour to achieve the desired outcomes. Whilst there may be collaboration and agreement of treatment plans and goals, the underlying premise is that the person has things 'done' to them by a powerful other. This is not what occurs in person-centred compassionate care.

Cognitive behavioural approaches to managing the therapeutic relationship

Cognitive behavioural approaches initially developed from the behavioural perspective in psychology. The approach of Pavlov and Skinner was seen to be too mechanistic and a shift occurred through the work of psychologists such as Thorndike and Bandura, leading to the cognitive perspective (see Chapter 1).

There have been a number of therapies developed in this area:

- Beck, in the 1960s, whose background was in psychoanalysis, focused on automatic negative thoughts and identified the cognitive triad leading to 'cognitive therapy'
- Ellis, from the 1960s to 1990s, whose background was in psychoanalysis, developed rational emotive therapy, which became 'rational emotive behavioural therapy' and established the ABC model (in this case: A = activating, B = beliefs, C = consequences)
- Bandura, in the 1960s and 1970s, developed social learning theory, which established 'social behavioural therapy'

General principles of cognitive behavioural approaches

- Cognition effects behaviour and emotions
- Cognition can be accessed and changed
- Behaviour can be changed
- Behaviour affects cognition and emotions

According to cognitive theory people undertake an activity called 'reasoning' where their interaction with the world is through a process of interpretation and inference. Due to distorted interpretations and 'inferences' people's reasoning is said to become faulty. This can lead to reasoning becoming biased and rigid and this can be **self-perpetuating**. Cognitive theory and associated therapies identify that these underlying distortions of reasoning can be accessed and changed.

The underlying assumptions of cognitive therapies are that each person has unique experiences of the world which leads to a unique way of interpreting the world. Through these, people **construct** their view of the world and their own belief system. People then go on to act on these beliefs and interpretations. They also collect information to support their beliefs and ways of interpreting the world.

Cognitive therapies are frequently provided alongside behavioural therapies and are called 'cognitive behavioural therapy' (CBT) as it is assumed that there is an interrelationship between thoughts, feelings and behaviour. CBT involves both **cognitive restructuring** and changing behaviours through classical, operant and social learning identified above. These therapists recognise the importance of association, reinforcement, beliefs and automatic thoughts (self-talk).

Cognitive behavioural therapy is based on developing new adaptive learning, which will address the automatic thoughts and presenting behaviours. The therapist will endeavour to use the following approaches:

- Problem-solving
- Focusing on the present
- Supporting self-efficacy
- Explicit goal-setting
- Collaboration

Most care practitioners will not become cognitive behavioural therapists but problem-solving, supporting self-efficacy, goal-setting and collaboration can all be part of their undertaking. The care practitioner using a person-centred compassionate approach would not present themselves as a therapist or expert. They would use their warmth and communication skills to enhance the individual's strengths to achieve their personal goals.

Some of the techniques used by CBT therapists could also be useful to care practitioners, such as helping the person to build skills like assertiveness and progressive relaxation.

Cognitive behavioural therapies have continued to grow from the early work of Beck, Ellis and Bandura. The current third wave of cognitive behavioural therapies focus more on the affective component of distress, and Marsha Linehan can be seen as the first of these approaches. Linehan developed dialectical behavioural therapy in the 1980s focusing on helping people with borderline personality disorder. Hayes, Strosahl and Wilson developed acceptance and commitment therapy in the 1990s, and then mindfulness-based cognitive therapy (MBCT) was developed in early 2000s through the work of Segal, Williams and Teasdale, followed by compassion-focused therapy (CFT) in the mid to late 2000s by Gilbert.

Dialectical behavioural therapy (DBT)

Dialectical behavioural therapy (DBT) accepts the cognitive therapeutic approach and collaboration identified above but also includes additional support in terms of helping the person find their strengths. Linehan (1993a), who developed this therapy, writes that people with emotional dysregulation such as borderline personality disorder have a **biological predisposition** and have experienced an **invalidating environment** whilst young. This leads to an increased vulnerability to health problems.

DBT is a specialised therapy that is used by extensively trained therapists but it can support the care practitioner's understanding and offer some support for their compassionate care.

Through their youth, people with these mental health problems develop dysfunctional assumptions about the world and this leads to their engagement in unhelpful **dialectics**. They tend to display dialectics of extreme emotional outburst or inhibition, and active passivity or apparent competence, positioning themselves at one end of the pole or the other instead of somewhere along the continuum.

Therapy aims to replace these dialectics with a more helpful one called 'acceptance and change'. This facilitates the person's acceptance of themselves and their circumstances but also to work towards change. It is provided through individual weekly sessions with a DBT therapist and weekly group sessions which are skills-based. The skills are categorised as:

- *Interpersonal effectiveness*: Through objective effectiveness, relationship effectiveness and self-respect
- *Distress tolerance/reality acceptance*: Through self-soothing, distraction and making the moment the best it can be
- *Emotion regulation*: By reducing vulnerability, increasing abilities and building positive experiences
- *Mindfulness*: Through the person experiencing their body, mind and world in the here and now (Linehan, 1993b)

The individual sessions include strategies of:

- *Eliciting goals*: What is it that the person would like to achieve for themselves?
- *Identifying values*: What is important to the person?
- *Developing commitment*: Through exploring the pros and cons of change; availability of choice
- *Validation*: The therapist acknowledging the person's experiences and how they feel about these

All these strategies and techniques can be useful in any therapeutic relationship. They can all be seen to be person-centred and offer compassion.

Acceptance and commitment therapy (ACT)

This therapy can be seen to be very similar to CBT and DBT but, instead of focusing on problems to develop goals to control themselves, the aim is to create a rich and meaningful life. This, it is believed, is achieved by just noticing what is occurring and accepting it. People are encouraged to recognise all their experiences, both the good and the bad, and to accept that both happen.

As with DBT, acceptance and commitment therapy (ACT) clarifies the values held by the person and teaches them skills. ACT uses acceptance and mindfulness strategies, together with commitment and behaviour change strategies, to increase psychological flexibility.

It has six core processes:

- Awareness of and focus on the present
- Cognitive defusion – to honestly identify experiences
- Acceptance – allowing thoughts and feelings to come and go
- Observing self – recognising who and what the self is for the person
- Values – to identify personal values and use these to guide behaviour
- Committed action – deciding what is important and working towards that

Mindfulness-based cognitive therapy (MBCT)

Activity 7.4   Mindfulness experience

Find somewhere comfortable to sit or lie down. Try to empty your mind by focusing on your body and all its sensations. Work slowly through your body:

- Do any of your muscles feel tense? Relax them.
- Do you have physical discomfort? Move until you feel more comfortable.
- What can you hear? Are the sounds from outside or inside your body? Recognise these sounds as demonstration that you are alive.
- What can you smell? What memories does this provoke?
- Do you have any other bodily sensations?
- Now think about somewhere you felt warm, comfortable and accepted. As you go about your normal tasks, if things become tense or stressful, take your mind back to this place.

An outline explanation can be found at the end of the chapter.

Mindfulness-based cognitive therapy (MBCT) adopts CBT's underlying assumptions about the person and therapeutic techniques but also engages mindfulness strategies. It was developed for people who experienced repeated or long-term depression.

The core processes for MBCT are:

- Self-awareness – thoughts, feelings, etc.
- To become in touch with feeling alive
- To halt escalation – to stop the downward spiral into depression
- Developing an alternative mode of mind by experiencing the world directly, non-conceptually and non-judgementally
- Supporting the recognition and experiencing of difficult emotions and thoughts

Compassion-focused therapy (CFT)

Compassion-focused therapy (CFT) is another of the third-wave cognitive behavioural approaches to therapy (MacBeth and Gumley, 2012) for people struggling with their well-being. Paul Gilbert (2009) developed a model of compassion (see Chapter 4) based on the interaction of biology, psychology and spirituality (namely Buddhism) within an evolutionary context. This understanding of compassion and self-shame led to his development of CFT.

Gilbert (2009) suggests that people have developed, evolutionarily, a threat/protection system, a **drive system** and a contentment system. If these are balanced, the person will maintain their well-being. It is when these are unbalanced that the person will develop problems. There is a strong interrelationship between the threat protection system and the drive system, which can motivate the person to deal with fearful or dysfunctional thoughts in an overactive manner. This might not be a problem if the contentment system is functioning well, but if it is not, the person has high levels of stress without the ability to self-soothe – show self-compassion. Lack of self-compassion has been found to have a significant impact on well-being (MacBeth and Gumley, 2012).

The core processes for CFT are:

- The therapist uses the skills of and expresses compassion
- The person will experience all of the attributes of compassion from the therapist
- The therapist helps the person develop skills and attributes for self-compassion

Case study

Imad Al Din

Imad Al Din was admitted to the medical unit complaining of severe lower abdominal pain, nausea and difficulty in urination. Several routine blood and physical assessments were performed and the results showed that the patient had prostate cancer. The policy in this hospital was that physicians (no other professionals) within the treatment team must disclose the diagnosis and break the news for any urgent or treatment-related decisions, options or findings. One of the team's physicians was available in the unit and decided to deliver the news, despite not having spoken with Imad Al Din before. The physician went to Imad Al Din's room and found that he was attended by his grandson, who was in his mid-20s. He asked Imad Al Din's grandson if he would like him to share their findings with him. Imad Al Din naively told the physician to speak out and tell him. The physician quickly and concisely explained that Imad Al Din had prostate cancer and that he needed treatment for this. Imad Al Din was unprepared for this information and had a limited knowledge of hospitals and medicine, and so started crying. Imad Al Din thought he was going to die and told the physician that he did not accept their test results. The grandson started shouting at the physician and aggressively telling him to leave the room. The physician ignored the grandson and continued to try to explain his position and the urgent need for him to break the news.

In the case study of Imad Al Din, we can see that the physician, patient (Imad Al Din) and his grandson are not demonstrating a balance between the evolutionary systems of threat/protection, drive (motivation) and contentment. Imad Al Din's threat/protection system has become more powerful as he tries to manage the information that has been shared with him. The physician also is struggling with his threat/protection system as can be seen by his need to explain himself. The grandson likewise has a more active threat/ protection system as indicated by his aggressive communication with the physician.

All of them are also failing to manage to self-soothe to support their contentment system. We can therefore see all of their behaviour driven or motivated towards aggression rather than assertion.

The physician is motivated by his desire to cure (the role of the physician) and his need to protect himself. From a spiritual and humanistic perspective, he is responding to his own value systems rather than the life world of the patient. Using the CFT approach, the physician needs to demonstrate *sensitivity and sympathy* to Imad Al Din as a person and his current situation. A focus on *well-being* rather than cure would assist the physician in finding out what is important for Imad Al Din so that he shows *warmth, empathy and a non-judgemental* approach. Within the current situation, the attribute of *distress tolerance* will help the physician to put on one side the threat he feels and stop his self-protection behaviour.

The attributes of compassion are:

- Sensitivity
- Sympathy
- Distress tolerance
- Empathy
- Non-judgement
- Care for well-being

In the case study of Imad Al Din, the physician could use the skills indicated below to develop a compassion-focused management of his relationship to enhance well-being of both patient and grandson.

The skills of demonstrating compassion in this situation are:

- *Compassionate attention*: The physician could focus on Imad Al Din's positive qualities, developing their appreciation and gratitude for these
- *Compassionate reasoning*: The physician needs to facilitate exploration of the evidence for thoughts such as 'I am going to die' and behaviours such as crying and shouting, seeking alternative understandings with a focus on kindness, support and helpfulness
- *Compassionate behaviour*: The physician could support them in facing the feared situation (exposure) with encouragement whilst focusing on developing positive processing of the situation
- *Compassionate sensation*: Encouraging the grandfather and grandson to recognise how compassion feels bodily through their thoughts and behaviours of kindness, support and warmth
- *Compassionate feeling*: The physician could help them develop thoughts and images that self-soothe
- *Compassionate imagery*: To imagine what self-compassion is like and how that feels

Summary

Whilst most care practitioners will not become specialised therapists, an exploration of the historical development of empirical talking therapies is useful for understanding the principles underpinning the techniques used to assess their credibility and ethic. There are a few techniques that are transferable such as relaxation, mindfulness, validating the person and problem-solving (Table 7.1).

Table 7.1 Overview of therapeutic approaches

Therapy	Developers	Role of therapist	Role of client
Classical conditioning	Pavlov	Manipulate the environment – develop associations	Passive recipient
Operant conditioning	Skinner	Manipulate the environment – punishment/reward	Passive recipient
Social learning	Bandura	Manipulate the environment – provide learning opportunity	Attends to role model
Cognitive behavioural therapy	Beck/Ellis	Educator	Active involvement
Dialectical behavioural therapy	Linehan	Educator/facilitator/validator	Active involvement
Acceptance and commitment therapy	Hayes et al.	Educator/facilitator/validator	Active involvement
Mindfulness	Segal et al.	Facilitator/validator	Active involvement/ self-management
Compassion-focused therapy	Gilbert	Carer/facilitator/educator	Active involvement/ self-management/self-compassion

Behavioural approaches to therapeutic engagement and relationships started from the therapist being 'in control' and manipulating the environment to facilitate change in a person's behaviour. This was then developed through a cognitive shift, recognising that people did not just respond to stimuli but that they also processed information from the environment. This led to a cognitive behavioural approach to therapeutic interventions. The third wave of cognitive behavioural therapies developed a more affective-focused approach. This third wave moved to focus on compassion, including not only cognition, behaviour and affect, but also a spiritual element which can be seen in the humanistic perspective in psychology.

Humanistic approaches to managing the therapeutic relationship

The humanistic perspective is not just one organised theory, but is based on a number of principles, from psychoanalytic and behavioural thought to the philosophical thoughts of phenomenology, particularly existentialism (see Chapters 1 and 5).

Existential philosophy

Existential philosophy's premises are that an individual is:

- Unique
- Aware of their life world experiences
- Able to control their experiences
- Free to make their own choices
- Responsible for their own existence

Existential philosophy formed the basis for humanistic psychology and the basis for the development of humanistic philosophy.

The principles of humanistic philosophy:

- Each person has control over their behaviour and experiences
- People are aware of their own life world experiences
- On the path to self-actualisation the person is always in the process of becoming something different
- Each person has the responsibility to realise their own potential
- People who refuse to become will not realise the full possibilities of human existence
- Consciousness, subjective feelings, moods and personal experiences are crucial because they all relate to one's existence in the world

This philosophy underpinned the theories of all the humanistic theorists. Whilst Maslow was considered the first humanistic psychologist, the leading proponent of this approach was Carl Ransom Rogers (1902–87). Rogers, as with the other humanistic psychologists, was influenced by theorists such as Freud, Thorndike and John Dewey, but he was also influenced by his own childhood deprivation.

From his theory about the person, Rogers developed a therapy called 'client-centred therapy' that was later to be recognised as 'person-centred therapy'. His underlying theory of the person had a number of assumptions, which were:

- Each person has their own sense of reality which is called their phenomenological field; this develops through their experiences of the world
- Each person has a self-actualising tendency that motivates them to achieve their potential: self-actualisation
- Each person is continually undergoing an organismic valuing process – placing more value on experiences that move them towards self-actualisation

Given the above assumptions, it can be seen that within client-centred therapy there is the need for clients to understand their self (self-concept) to enable them to continue towards their potential or to self-actualise. These will be unique as each phenomenological field or life world is different.

Rogers (1951) identified that the way people view themselves could be congruent or incongruent. 'Incongruent' implies that the self-concept is based on **conditions of worth** rather than the organismic valuing process. Conditions of worth are where people place a higher value on achieving positive regard from others, rather than the attainment of personal potential: self-actualisation. Positive regard is necessary for a congruent self-concept but to strive for this in some sense devalues it, as to support self-concept it needs to be unconditional. Despite the problems of actively seeking positive regard, the person, through a process of **subception** and **defence**, protects incongruence and prevents change (Rogers, 1951). They offer explanations and rationales for why it is important to do things to please others and gain positive regard from them.

Within client-centred therapy, person-centred therapy and all humanistic approaches to therapy, there are four core conditions which the therapist must achieve:

- Empathy
- Genuineness or congruence
- Warmth
- Unconditional positive regard

Empathy

This is the ability to understand the other person's feelings and to be able to demonstrate this understanding to them. It is the ability to step inside the phenomenological field or life world of the other person – to perceive their reality as they do, to sense, feel and understand the personal meanings of their experience:

> Empathy is to feel 'with'. Sympathy is to feel 'like'. Pity is to feel 'for'. (Stewart, 2005: 108)

Genuineness or congruence

This is to do with being 'real'. It is not behaving in a certain way because it is believed that is the way that care practitioners should behave, but behaving in a way that the individual feels is right. It is about being true to oneself or 'comfortable in one's own skin'. It is what is being sought for by the person in distress and being demonstrated by the therapist.

Warmth

Warmth can be demonstrated through both verbal and non-verbal communication. Soft, calm and slow use of verbal language alongside a relaxed, open and attentive body posture can show warmth. This enables the relationship to develop through a feeling of comfort and it can encourage trust.

Unconditional positive regard

This is the fundamental attitude needed when working with people using a Rogerian approach. There is the need to feel positively towards the other person regardless of anything they may say or do. This is the core need for people. People have psychological problems because they have not received this in childhood and therefore do not have a positive self-regard. The care practitioner needs to be consistently accepting of the person demonstrating warmth.

 Halim Al Qatar

Halim is 20 years old and was diagnosed with thalassaemia. He has had many admissions to hospital but usually to the high-dependency section of a female medical unit so that his mother can continue to care for him. He lives in a culture that does permit men and women in the same hospital units. His mother does not allow him to undertake any daily living activities without her involvement. The patient does not initiate conversation with anybody else during his admission and usually covers his face so he that does not need to respond whenever approached. The mother has always refused the admission of her son to the male unit as she was concerned about his safety. Therefore, he was admitted to the female unit so she could stay with him and continue supporting him. However, the female patients at the unit and the female staff started complaining about having a male patient on the unit.

The nursing officer at the hospital reviewed the situation and decided to move Halim to a male unit. His mother was informed of the decision and staff came to move him, escorted by the nursing officer. The mother had refused to consent to the move, despite the explanations of the staff and started to become verbally abusive.

During the interactions, the nursing officer observed that the mother was unaware of her son's current health status; she believed he should not mix with other patients. After arriving on the male unit, the mother started becoming physically abusive towards the nursing officer. Halim had not been involved in the decision-making and did not show any reactions towards the situation. Finally, the mother started crying and broke down, indicating that no one understood and her feelings were not being considered. The nursing officer took the mother to a private room to further discuss the situation with her.

Through attentive listening and positive encouragement, the nursing officer came to understand that the mother had many family issues and that she was not being supported. Halim's father and brother were not involved in his care as they did not feel able. The mother had not been approached before this incident to identify Halim's personal and social situation. Therefore, Halim and his mother had quietly just accepted it. The nursing officer organised that Halim's father and brother were given the health education they needed and became involved in the treatment. The involvement of male members of his family and his mother's reduced responsibility had a positive effect on Halim and his mother.

An exploration of the case study of Halim can facilitate an understanding of the importance of using a person-centred approach. This scenario occurred in a culture where there was clear delineation between men and women but, despite the cultural differences, the principles of person-centred communication are still essential for high-quality care. In the case study, the nursing officer managed a difficult situation according to hospital policies and religious and cultural expectations but this left the mother distraught. Given the mother's behaviour, she could have been ordered to leave the hospital but the nursing officer recognised that she is only concerned for her son. Whilst aggressive behaviour cannot be condoned, the nursing officer has attempted to demonstrate *understanding* (*empathy*) and *warmth* towards the mother, despite her behaviour. The mother was also taken to a private space thereby maintaining her dignity.

Using person-centred communication (*positive regard, non-judgemental approach*) the nursing officer was able to have a better understanding of Halim's situation and facilitate his growth as well as his mother's well-being whilst still upholding her own values: *congruence*.

Summary

The Rogerian approach to the therapeutic relationship is focused on the relationship, whereas cognitive and behavioural approaches focus on the therapy or skills. Rogerian client-centred therapy has become the basis for communication education for care professionals.

Gerard Egan's skilled helper

Gerard Egan, Professor of Organization Studies and Psychology at Loyola University, Chicago, developed a model of skilled helping: this is a three-stage model. Egan's therapeutic approach is from within the humanistic approach but he, unlike Rogers, recognised the need for some boundaries and goal-setting within the counselling relationship and chose to call his approach 'skilled helping'.

Egan's three-stage model of helping

1. Review the current scenario
2. Develop the preferred scenario
3. Formulation of action plans (Egan, 1977)

Review the current scenario

This stage is where the person is enabled to tell their story, using the same therapeutic relationship identified by Rogers. This is a collaborative approach where the listener uses **reflection, paraphrasing** and **echoing**. This enables them to highlight **blind spots** in the story, facilitating a wider understanding of the problems they are trying to overcome. The helper challenges the person to own their problems and opportunities and to state problems as solvable, recognising they may be faulty interpretations. The person will also be supported to search for **leverage**, which is searching for a reason, to overcome the problem. If there is no leverage, then there is no reason to deal with the problem.

Developing the desired scenario

The person is helped to identify what they would prefer their situation to be: their desired scenario. Within Egan's therapy, a goal is needed so that what is being working towards is established. Identification of the preferred scenario allows the development of objectives and goals. The person needs to commit to these changes in order to achieve the desired scenario.

Formulation of action plans

At this stage, the goals identified in the previous stage are transformed into an action plan. With assistance, the person may use a number of strategies to achieve this such as brainstorming, **divergent thinking** and thinking creatively. The plans need to include sub-goals along with contingency plans. The person will need support and to establish things to maintain their motivation. Egan writes that there is the need for evaluation and feedback throughout the process to ensure success.

Alongside a staged helping process, Egan also offers care practitioners practice skills to engagement, support and develop the therapeutic process. These are through verbal and non-verbal communication skills.

Therapeutic communication skills

Throughout this chapter, an exploration of psychological theory has led to different approaches to helping people in distress through the therapies associated with them. To be effective in all of the therapies considered, fundamentally there is the need to:

*   Listen
*   Attend
*   Respond

If a care practitioner is unable to do these, then they will be unable to develop a therapeutic relationship.

Egan (1977) offers a basic format for listening and attending in his book *The Skilled Helper* (Figure 7.3):

- S – sit squarely; this means sitting up-right and alert
- O – open posture; crossing arms and legs may appear to be a barrier
- L – lean forward; how far forward will depend on what is being said: if the person is distressed leaning forward could be a sign of concern but if the person is agitated or anxious it may feel like an invasion of their personal space
- E – eye contact; a consistent gaze is important but should not be constant as this could indicate disapproval
- R – relax; if you appear relaxed and confident this may reassure the person

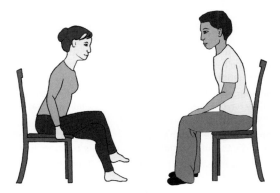

Figure 7.3   SOLER

Stickley (2011) further developed this format for sitting and attending to a person, and identified the following technique (Figure 7.4):

- S – sit at an angle
- U – uncross arms and legs
- R – relax
- E – eye contact
- T – touch
- Y – your intuition

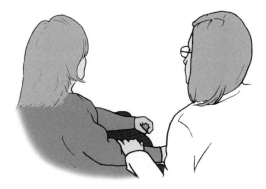

Figure 7.4   SURETY

Whilst there are many similarities between the two formats, Stickley encourages a more congruent approach giving the caregiver permission to respond in a genuine way using their intuition rather than conforming to guidelines. He also recognises the importance of touch within therapeutic interactions. There will be cultural differences in proximity, amount of eye contact, touch and body posture between and within groups, particularly gender groups as was seen in the case study of Halim, and these need to form part of using 'your intuition'.

Egan (1977) also offers information on how to respond within caregiving relationships (Table 7.2).

Table 7.2   Types of responding identified by Egan (1977)

Verbal responding	Non-verbal responding
The appropriate use of open (for encouraging the person to talk) and closed questions (such as when the person is confused or in pain and information is needed)	Postural echoing (taking up the same posture as the patient or client)
Reflecting (demonstrating empathetic understanding by inwardly digesting what they have said, offering it back to them in a different verbal format)	Nodding (to demonstrate agreement and that what has been said has been heard and accepted)
Paraphrasing (brief response using the person's own words may condense and clarify the information)	Smiling (to demonstrate warmth and encouragement)
Echoing (stating the last sentence the person has said to encourage further explanation)	Touch (this is dependent on the person's need for personal space but holding hands or touching forearms can demonstrate empathy)
Summarising (offering a shortened version of what has been said including the main points)	Silence (sometimes the use of silence can be helpful to allow the person time to reflect but know you are still present and attending)

Whilst these are techniques that can be tried out when unsure, person-centred compassionate care is about being 'real' and showing care in a genuine manner. Lennart Fredriksson highlighted intersubjectivity and how this facilitated comfort. He described nurses using their presence, touch and listening to provide compassionate care (Fredriksson, 1999). Like Fredriksson, Dewar's conceptualisation of compassionate relationship-centred care, which is underpinned by communication, identifies the need for 'appreciative caring conversations' (Dewar, 2011, cited Dewar and Nolan, 2013: 1248).

The effective therapeutic relationship

Stewart (2005) says that the therapeutic relationship is influenced by:

- How the core conditions of empathy, genuineness, non-possessive warmth and unconditional positive regard are demonstrated
- The experience of trust, feeling safe and having faith in the caregiver
- The style of interaction of both people
- The way in which transference and countertransference are acknowledged and worked through

Stewart can be seen to have an eclectic approach to the therapeutic relationship, accepting elements from differing perspectives. Care practitioners may find the same approach most useful. In order to address the influencing factors above, there is initially a need to develop self-awareness.

Chapter summary

This chapter has considered each of the psychological perspectives and explored therapies that have developed from each of them. All therapies can offer care practitioners some guidance on how to manage their therapeutic relationships. To increase self-awareness, which is seen as essential for all therapeutic approaches, is considered an ongoing process throughout the care career.

Further study

The British Association of Behavioural and Cognitive Psychotherapies website offers information on this therapeutic approach, evidence for its efficacy and how to access training. See: www.babcp.com/About/About.aspx

The British Psychoanalytic Council website offers information about psychoanalytic/psychodynamic therapies, the evidence to support the approach and how to access training. See: www.bpc.org.uk/

Activity outline answer

Activity 7.4   Mindfulness experience

Taking time to undertake an exercise similar to this one allows the opportunity to focus on the present, taking time out from the stress of what has been done and what might yet occur. It allows you to relax your muscles and be aware of and accept yourself, your thoughts, feelings and sensations. Mindfulness can create a feeling of peace and help you recognise when you are becoming anxious, worried or stressed in the future and reduce this before it becomes a health problem.

References

Bandura, A. (1977) *Social Learning Theory*. Upper Saddle River, NJ: Prentice Hall.

Barker, S. (2007) *Vital Notes for Nurses: Psychology*. Oxford: Blackwell.

Dewar, B. and Nolan, M. (2013) 'Caring about caring: Developing a model to implement compassionate relationship-centred care in an older-people care setting', *International Journal of Nursing Studies*, 50 (9): 1247–58.

Egan, G. (1977) *The Skilled Helper*. Monterey, CA: Brooks/Cole.

Fredriksson, L. (1999) 'Modes of relating in a caring conversation: A research synthesis on presence, touch and listening', *Journal of Advanced Nursing*, 30 (5): 1167–76.

Gilbert, P. (2009) 'Introducing compassion-focused therapy', *Advances in Psychiatric Treatment*, 15: 199–208.

Lazarus, R.S. (1966) *Psychological Stress and the Coping Process*. New York: McGraw-Hill.

Linehan, M.M. (1993a) *Cognitive-Behavioural Treatment of Borderline Personality Disorder*. London: Guilford Press.

Linehan, M.M. (1993b) *Skills Training Manual for Treating Borderline Personality Disorder*. London: Guilford Press.

Luft, J. and Ingham, H. (1955) 'The Johari Window: A graphic model of interpersonal awareness', in J. Luft (1969), *Of Human Interaction: The Johari Model*. Palo Alto, CA: National Press, p. 170.

MacBeth, A. and Gumley, A. (2012) 'Exploring compassion: A meta-analysis of the association between self-compassion and psychopathology', *Clinical Psychology Review*, 32: 545–52.

Maslow, A. (1954) *Motivation and Personality*. New York: Harper and Row.

Pavlov, I. (1927) *Conditioned Reflexes*. London: Oxford University Press.

Rogers, C.R. (1951) *Client-Centred Therapy*. London: Constable.

Skinner, B.F. (1938) *The Behavior of Organisms: An Experimental Analysis*. Cambridge, MA: B.F. Skinner Foundation.

Stewart, W. (2005) *An A–Z of Counselling Theory and Practice*. Eastleigh: Nelson Thornes.

Stickley, T. (2011) 'From SOLER to SURETY for effective non-verbal communication', *Nurse Education in Practice*, 11: 395–8.

Thorndike, E.L. (1999 [1913]) *Education Psychology: Briefer Course*. New York: Routledge.

8 Emotional Intelligence

Sue Barker, Beverley Johnson and Andrew Santos

Socrates said (ThinkExist, 2015):

I know that I am intelligent, because I know that I know nothing.

Einstein (Goodreads, 2015) said:

The true sign of intelligence is not knowledge but imagination.

Learning objectives

Intelligence was one of the first areas psychologists started to explore over two hundred years ago. The concept has developed over this time and more recently the term has been developed to include emotional intelligence. Emotional intelligence is the focus of this chapter. This chapter's learning objectives are to:

- Describe intelligence
- Explore the social world in which emotional intelligence has become necessary
- Critically examine emotional intelligence

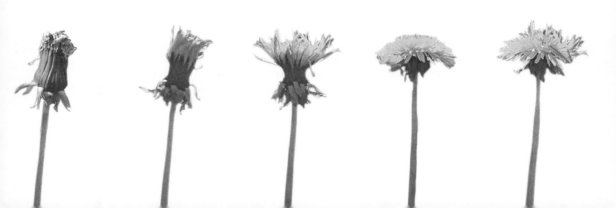

Activity 8.1   Critical thinking

Do you consider yourself to be intelligent? Do you think that it is necessary to be intelligent to be a good caregiver?

An outline answer can be found at the end of this chapter.

Intelligence

Intelligence appears to be highly valued within Western societies and there are numerous intelligence tests available. Since its inception as a psychological difference to be examined and measured, it has been seen to be a method for predicting who will do best in a given situation. Initially, there were two major approaches, one by Sir Francis Galton (1822–1911) and the other by Alfred Binet (1857–1911).

Francis Galton

Galton believed that intelligence consisted of two general qualities:

- *Strength*: Muscular strength, speed and accuracy in performing tasks
- *Psycho-biological ability*: Ability to see, hear, taste and touch accurately

He also believed that if these abilities were measured, they would indicate the intelligence level of the person and predict their future success. This is a biological view of intelligence, which would indicate that intelligence is due to inherited or genetic factors. These genetic factors could be developed through training. Galton's motivation to study intelligence was influenced by his belief in eugenics: he was one of the founders of the eugenics movement in Britain. This movement suggested that selective breeding would enhance the human species. Unfortunately for Galton, he was unable to provide evidence that his tests predicted future success. Whilst the early tests of the English scientist Galton did not correlate with real-life achievements, the work of the French scientist Binet went on to be influential in present-day intelligence tests.

Alfred Binet and Théodore Simon

Binet's motivation and view of intelligence was quite different to Galton's. The French Ministry of Education in early the 1900s asked him to develop tests in order to establish the abilities of children to predict and ensure their success. He did this in collaboration with Théodore Simon (1872–1961). The tests which they developed could identify high achievers as well as those with different levels of learning disability. The tests involved the children making judgements in which they demonstrated practical sense, adaptability and initiative. Unlike Galton, who assumed a biological view of intelligence, Binet's view was more similar to that of the behaviourists.

Activity 8.2   Example intelligence test questions similar to those used by Binet with children

1.   Question 1: Horse is to cart as engine is to . . .
2.   Question 2: Andrew is older than Peter and David is older than Andrew. Who is the youngest?
3.   Question 3: What comes next in the sequence 13243546?
4.   Question 4: Rearrange the letters *rapsi* to identify the city.

Answers are given at the end of the chapter.

Louis L. Thurstone: Primary mental abilities

Psychologist Louis L. Thurstone (1887–1955) developed a theory that focused on seven different 'primary mental abilities'. These he believed constituted intelligence leading to intelligent behaviour:

- Verbal comprehension
- Reasoning
- Perceptual speed
- Numerical ability
- Word fluency
- Associative memory
- Spatial visualisation

The abilities identified by Thurstone can be seen to link well with the current two established types of intelligence, which are:

- Crystallised intelligence
- Fluid intelligence

Crystallised intelligence

Crystallised intelligence is deemed to be experience dependent and involves abilities such as verbal comprehension (understanding what other people say), general information, experiential evaluation (judging something based on previous experience of it), remote verbal associations (identifying an association between words) and arithmetic skill (speeded).

Fluid intelligence

Fluid intelligence is associated with physiology. It is dependent on physiology abilities and can therefore be seen to deteriorate with age. Fluid intelligence involves the abilities of inductive reasoning (logical process of working through problems to arrive at an answer), figural reasoning (sometimes known as 'abstract reasoning', the ability to see patterns, trends; lateral thinking), unspeeded reasoning (when there is time to logically work through a problem,), visual organisation, common analogies and perceptual speed.

We can therefore see that both a biological readiness as well as an environmental stimulation can influence a person's ability to demonstrate intelligence. Since these types of intelligence were developed, further theories of intelligence were created in the 1980s but all of these theories recognised the importance of culture. Gardner (1983) developed a theory of multiple intelligences and Sternberg (1985) developed his triarchic theory.

Gardner's multiple intelligences

- *Linguistic*: The use of language, useful for passing on information and telling stories
- *Logical*: Mathematical – the ability to solve mathematical problems
- *Spatial*: The ability to recognise spatial differences, for example a diagram when it has been rotated, which can useful for driving vehicles
- *Musical*: The ability to sing, play an instrument or compose
- *Bodily*: Kinaesthetic – having a detailed understanding of where one's own body is can be useful in dancing and gymnastics
- *Interpersonal*: The ability to develop relationships with others
- *Intrapersonal*: The understanding of oneself: self-awareness
- *Naturalistic*: The understanding or ability to classify the natural world

Sternberg's triarchic intelligence

1. *Creative*: The ability to develop new ways of thinking, behaving and feeling
2. *Practical*: The ability to put knowledge and skills into practice
3. *Analytical*: The ability to solve problems

All of these theories recognise a contextual or cultural element in intellectual ability. It is therefore important that we consider the social world in which people need to demonstrate intelligence.

Summary

There are a number of theories of intelligence, including the dual biological one of crystallised and fluid intelligence, the more social theory of multiple intelligence and the cognitive theory of triarchic intelligence. Contemporary society generally accepts that there are a number of different types of intelligence as suggested by Gardner, but whilst they are all related to skills that could be performed, there is also an identification that all these skills need to grow and be demonstrated within the social world; they are influenced by culture and context.

Social world of compassionate care

Groups

Carlson et al. (2004: 659) define a group as: 'a collection of individuals who have a shared definition of who they are and what they should think, feel and do – people in the same group generally have common interests and goals'. Given this definition, we could view large collaborations such as government bodies as well as small collaborations such as family and friends to be groups.

The government, in numerous publications, have stressed the importance of all care services working together to provide optimal care and safeguard both children and adults. We are increasingly seeing large organisations such as the National Institute for Health and Care Excellence (NICE) collaborating with the Social Care Institute of Excellence (SCIE) to develop education and guidance. We have also seen the bringing-together of psychologists, occupational therapists, physiotherapists and operating department practitioners under the umbrella of the Health Professions Council (HPC).

Effective groups

An effective group needs to fulfil a number of criteria, which have been identified as:

- Interaction
- Interdependence
- Stability
- Sharing of goals
- Structure/group roles
- Perception: the member recognises themselves as being part of the group

To be an effective group, the first step will be the coming-together of individuals. The coming-together or the formation of a group was described by Tuckman in the 1960s.

Group formation

It is suggested that a life cycle approach is useful in understanding groups and that groups go through set stages in the process of development, maintenance or maturation and termination.

Stages in group life, developed by Tuckman (1965):

- *Forming*: The coming-together and getting to know each other and the group aims
- *Storming*: When the individuals are establishing how they can work together
- *Norming*: When roles, responsibilities and objectives are established
- *Performing*: When the group is getting on with achieving the aims

To these original stages of the group lifespan developed by Tuckman, a further stage has been added called 'adjourning or mourning' for when the group task has been completed. The group may go on to become a social group when this happens.

A key concept within group effectiveness is group **cohesion**. Cohesiveness can be seen as the extent to which a group fits or hangs together. If it is cohesive, then the individuals fit together closely. Festinger et al. (1950) developed a model suggesting that a '**field of forces**' influences group cohesiveness (see Figure 8.1).

Festinger et al.'s field of forces has similar elements to the six elements of an effective group identified at the beginning of this section They identify that if each of the members finds the group and its other members attractive and they can work well together with mutually dependent goals – this becomes the field of forces and the group will be cohesive. This cohesion will lead to behaviours such as continued membership and an acceptance of group values, roles and standards.

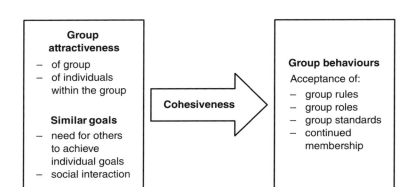

Figure 8.1   Field of forces

McGregor in 1960 went on to further explore group cohesiveness. He suggested that there were 11 factors that influenced group effectiveness:

- *Atmosphere*: Needs to be relaxed and comfortable
- *Discussion*: Should be focused and inclusive
- *Objectives*: Should be clear and accepted by all the group members
- *Listening*: All members should listen to one another, so that everyone feels free to express themselves
- *Disagreement*: The group should know how to deal with disagreement without avoidance
- *Decisions*: Should be made by consensus
- *Criticism*: This should be kept open and members should be able to accept constructive criticism
- *Feelings*: The members should able and willing to express their feelings
- *Action*: Should be clearly defined and all members fully committed
- *Leadership*: This should be flexible
- *Self-consciousness*: The group should be aware of its operational features, and reflect on its own operation

Activity 8.3   Critical thinking

Explore the 11 factors identified by McGregor by thinking about a group that you have been part of which have worked together well and one that has not worked well. Were there any differences in the number of McGregor's factors which you perceived?

An outline answer can be found at the end of the chapter.

Summary

Groups are extensively used within care through **informal** and **formal, multidisciplinary** and **inter-professional** groups. To be effective, these groups need to be cohesive, and to achieve this each member needs to feel attracted to the group and to the other members and they should have agreed goals. Each member should feel comfortable within the group and that they are an active member with a clear role to play.

Relationship theories

As can be seen from the previous sections of this chapter, interactions between people are crucial within care. Care, whilst usually an individual activity, needs to be organised either within a team or with team support. These teams or groups need to be cohesive. To achieve this, each of the group members should be attractive to each other and to the group. As stated, care is usually a one-to-one activity, so every carer needs to develop individual relationships as well as team-working skills. The therapeutic relationship was considered in more detail in Chapter 7, so other types of individual interactions are considered here.

Interpersonal relationships

On first meeting, people start to form impressions and judgements about each other. These judgements influence the type of relationship that ensues. These relationships can be seen as at least partly culturally determined. Western societies place emphasis on romantic relationships between two people but other cultures put emphasis on the extended family and responsibility. As identified, for groups to be cohesive, the members need to be attracted to each other and the group; the same is true for individual relationships. For individual relationships to be fulfilling, each person needs to find the relationship and the other person attractive.

Physical attractiveness

The first time that people meet, what will usually be noticed is what the person looks like, unless the observer has impaired vision. To be physically attractive is a great advantage as it offers the person more opportunities in life, although the perception of attractiveness of individuals is influenced by the environment. If a person is in a situation which increases their anxiety they may find those around them more attractive as demonstrated in the study by Dutton and Aron (1974) where men found women more attractive when anxiety was provoked. In some situations attractiveness can be increased by altering the environment; for example if there is low lighting pupils dilate, which is perceived by the observer as indicating attraction.

There are stereotypes of an attractive person having, for example, symmetrical facial features; a male body shape of the waist being 70 per cent of the width of shoulders; and of females having the waist 70 per cent of the size of the hips. This is also identified as the healthiest shape, indicating a higher fertility rate. Physical attractiveness can, however, be seen as culturally determined as it changes with time and from one racial group to another.

Along with physical attractiveness stereotypes, there are also psychological attractiveness stereotypes. It is assumed as part of this stereotype that an attractive person will be warm, sociable, friendly and successful in all areas and enjoy life, which can be seen to be similar to effective role models.

Proximity, familiarity, similarity and reciprocity

One theory of relationships provides a process from **proximity** to **reciprocity**. Proximity of another person may lead to relationship development whereas distance may lead to relationships ceasing. Proximity offers the opportunity to get to know one another and develop a relationship. **Familiarity** can be seen as part of the process towards attraction and leads on from proximity. Despite a myth suggesting that 'familiarity breeds contempt', psychologists have found that, as a person becomes more familiar, they are perceived as more comfortable to be with. The individuals get 'used to' each other and can be viewed in a similar way to 'habituation' in learning theory. Along with proximity and familiarity, **similarity** and reciprocity are also seen to be important in developing and maintaining relationships. If people have similar attitudes, beliefs and values they tend to find each other more attractive. Also, people tend to like others more if they believe that they are liked in return: the liking can be seen to be reciprocal.

Similarity can be seen as rewarding as it could lead to agreement, which can make it easier to communicate with the other person, create a basis for engaging in joint activities, and those who agree with us can increase our confidence. It has been said that most people are vain enough to believe that anyone who shares their views must be sensitive and praiseworthy. Similarity can also lead to reciprocity in the relationship as we assume that people with similar attitudes to ourselves will like us, resulting in us liking them.

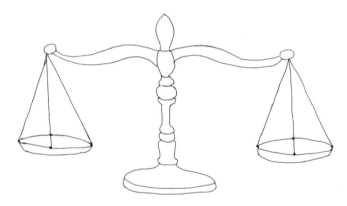

Figure 8.2   Balance scales

Social exchange theory

The social exchange theory is based on the reward approach of operant conditioning (behavioural perspective) but goes beyond this because it is interactional. Homans (1961) adapted the basic operant conditioning of Skinner to incorporate the following economic factors:

- *Cost reward ratio*: Working out what one has to give (cost) in a relationship in comparison to what one can get (reward)
- *Minimax strategy*: The concept that people try to give as little as possible for the greatest gain

- *Profit*: This is where the rewards (what is gained) exceed the costs (what has to be given)
- *Comparison level*: This is the standard by which other relationships are judged

Within a relationship, costs and rewards could be material, emotional, informational, services or status. This theory suggests that people are not altruistic but they are attempting to gain as much as possible, and whether a relationship works is dependent on each person believing that they are gaining an appropriate reward for their efforts. This can clearly be seen in recent Western societies where there is a focus on equity within relationships. The expectation is that there should be no profit but that each person should make the same effort and receive the same level of rewards.

Interestingly, despite there being an expectation of equity of effort within a partnership or marriage, this is in direct opposition to the stereotypes of love which identify love as selfless, forgiving, altruistic, a gift. In fact, the Christian religious text in the Bible (NIV, I Cor. 13:4–7), tells us:

> Love is patient, love is kind. It does not envy, it does not boast, it is not proud. It is not rude, it is not self-seeking, it is not easily angered, it keeps no record of wrongs. Love does not delight in evil but rejoices with the truth. It always protects, always trusts, always hopes, always perseveres. Love never fails.

The Qur'an likewise offers an understanding of love (Hubb) as being pure (2:222), involving sacrifice (2:177), not decaying (49:12) and being steadfast (3:146). Both of these religious texts do, however, identify God as being love, and those who are faithful to him being rewarded.

Theories of love

The development and maintenance of relationships as described above account for any type of relationship. Some would suggest that different types of relationship have different meanings and therefore differing explanations are needed. Certainly there are many texts that identify that professional caring relationships are different from informal relationships.

Hogg and Vaughan (1998: 467) offer a definition of two types of love:

- *Passionate (or romantic) love*: A state of intense absorption in another person involving physiological arousal
- *Companionate love*: Caring and affection for another person which usually arises from sharing time together

Activity 8.4   Critical thinking

Do you think that all loving relationships can be divided into these two categories?

An outline answer can be found at the end of the chapter.

Sternberg (2000) offers a triangular theory of love, which incorporates eight types of love but each type depends on the presence of the three basic components: intimacy, passion and commitment:

- *Intimacy* refers to a closeness or connection with another person within which thoughts, feeling and hopes are shared
- *Passion* is the desire, an intense erotic attraction, to unite with another person
- *Commitment* is the intention or decision to stay within a relationship

Sternberg's theory gives eight types of love which are dependent on whether intimacy, passion or commitment are part of the relationship:

- *Non-love* is where there is no intimacy, passion or commitment
- *Infatuated love* is where there is only passion
- *Liking (friendship)* is where there is only intimacy
- *Empty love* is where there is only commitment
- *Romantic love* is where there is passion and intimacy
- *Companionate love* is where there is intimacy and commitment
- *Fatuous love* contains only passion and commitment
- *Consummate love* has all three basic components: passion, intimacy and commitment

Sternberg suggests that people develop their own personal love stories and that loving relationships only develop when another person is found to take on the fantasised role. Both individuals need to fulfil the fantasised role of the other and as long as they do this then the relationship continues, whatever type of love the story holds.

An understanding of love relationships is important for caring givers as it is established that they have a profound impact on people and their sense of well-being. People who lost their love partner were much more likely than other people of the same age to die, as bereavement of a loved one has a huge impact on physical and mental health (Buckley et al., 2012). Children who lost one of their parents in their early years were twice as likely to die in early adulthood as those without this bereavement (Li et al., 2014). Whilst it is generally acknowledged that loving relationships are important for people, there is debate over whether a formal caring relationship should include the experience of loving.

In Chapter 4, we saw that care theorists were able to recognise love as a component of caring activities but many within Western cultures are unhappy with this inclusion, suggesting that it is 'overstepping' professional boundaries. Stickley and Freshwater (2002) offer an exploration of these issues within care

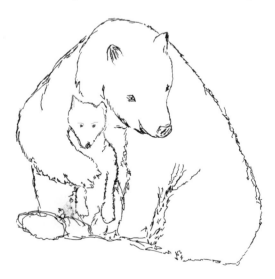

Figure 8.3 Polar bear and dog playing together

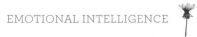

practice and firmly conceive of love as an important facet of a caring relationship, whether formal or informal.

Summary

There are a number of theories that help us explore relationships with others. These include: biological, such as the theory of physical attraction; cognitive, such as the proximity, familiarity, similarity and reciprocity theory and the social exchange theory; and emotional, the theories of love. Love can be seen as an emotional engagement with another person in which care and compassion can be demonstrated. If, as Stickley and Freshwater (2002) identify, it is essential in all caring relationships, then the ability to manage our emotions and the emotions of others is crucial to use love to support our care.

Activity 8.5 Reflection

Take some time to think about love and what it means to you.

Do you think it is an important part of your care provision?

As this is a reflection, there is no outline answer at the end of the chapter.

Read the case study of Mrs Jones and consider if there is a loving relationship between her and the nurse.

 ## Mrs Jones

Mrs Jones was a 64-year-old widow admitted to an acute medical ward. She was admitted with symptoms of lethargy, breathlessness and peripheral oedema. She was under the care of the general medical physicians and had been diagnosed with congestive cardiac failure.

Mrs Jones had been in hospital three days before I took over her care. During the nursing handover, it was highlighted that Mrs Jones was refusing all medical intervention and had requested to be allowed to die. Mrs Jones was therefore not for resuscitation. She was accepting personal care, but refused to get out of bed and wanted to go home to be with her family and to die in her own home. Nurses on the ward had begun to organise a care package for her discharge, involving the social worker and the district nurse planning together with family.

Mrs Jones had been offered psychological support from a counsellor, but had declined this. Capacity was not in question, and therefore the nurses on the ward had respected her wishes.

(Continued)

Case study

(Continued)

On introducing myself to Mrs Jones, I offered her assistance with her hygiene needs. Suggesting she might like to have a bath, I took the opportunity to wash and style her hair, massage moisturiser into her limbs and put make-up on her face.

This normal interaction allowed me to talk to Mrs Jones about her feelings and concerns. I initially asked why she wanted to go home to die and she stated that she knew that her condition was terminal, and that she was lonely and didn't see any point in postponing the inevitable. She intimated that her husband had died of the same and she didn't want the same undignified painful death that he had been exposed to.

I explored this somewhat further by asking where he had been when he was diagnosed, where he had died and what was offered to him in terms of treatment and palliative care. Tearfully, she informed me that he went into hospital with a chest infection and it was discovered that he had lung cancer. A lobectomy was performed and he spent two weeks acutely unwell in ITU (intensive treatment unit) with 'tubes coming out of him everywhere, and machines keeping him alive'. Following recovery from this acute event, he was then transferred to a ward for chemotherapy. During his time in hospital, whilst receiving chemotherapy, he developed 'complications' and deteriorated. The staff wanted to transfer him to ITU again, but the family refused. According to Mrs Jones, he died in hospital, confused and in pain and gasping for breath.

During this discussion, we talked about how she remembered her husband and she shared happy memories. I considered whether she understood what her condition was and asked about her understanding. She explained that she thought her symptoms of breathlessness were similar to her husband's and she didn't want to go through the same process: 'They wouldn't treat an animal like that.' When I advised her that she didn't have cancer and that she had heart failure that could be treated with medication, and that she could actually leave hospital reasonably well and actually function, she was astonished. I explained that she did have a cardiac condition but that she wasn't dying of cancer: her condition wasn't reversible but manageable. She hadn't for a second considered that she didn't have cancer. She very quickly consented to receiving active treatment and was keen to mobilise and be discharged home as well as she could possibly be.

Behaving towards Mrs Jones in a loving way through personal hygiene allowed Mrs Jones to express her concerns and the nurse to be able to clarify the situation, leading to a positive outcome for the care staff as well as for Mrs Jones and her family. Whether we call this type of care a 'loving relationship' or not, we can see that this type of compassionate care is working with the emotions of the person. The next section explores emotional intelligence, but theories of emotion and **emotion work** will also be explored in the next chapter (see Chapter 9).

Emotional intelligence (EI)

At the beginning of this chapter, we considered what intelligence was and recognised that it is difficult to define and that there are a number of theories of intelligence. It is generally accepted that there are a number of different types of intelligence as suggested by Gardner, but whilst they are all related to skills that could be performed, there was also an identification that all these skills need to grow and be demonstrated in the social world: they were influenced by culture and context.

The concept of 'emotional intelligence' (EI) can be seen to have grown from one of Gardner's types of intelligence, specifically interpersonal intelligence. Following on from this, in 1989 Peter Salovey and John Mayer developed a model of emotional intelligence. Daniel Goleman was to make this a global term with his bestselling book, *Emotional Intelligence: Why it Can Matter More than IQ*.

Mayer and Salovey (1997: 10) defined emotional intelligence as: the ability to perceive accurately, appraise and express emotion; the ability to access and or generate feelings when they facilitate thought; the ability to understand emotion and emotional knowledge; and the ability to regulate emotions to promote emotional and intellectual growth.

Mixed model of emotional intelligence

Emotional intelligence involves abilities and traits. It is a mixture of innate traits and learned abilities, which can be categorised into five domains (Goleman, 1995):

1. *Self-awareness*

   Observing yourself and recognising a feeling as it happens

2. *Managing one's own emotions or self-regulation*

   Handling feelings so that they are appropriate

   Realising what is behind a feeling

   Finding ways to handle fears and anxieties, anger and sadness

3. *Motivation of oneself*

   Channelling emotions in the service of a goal

   Emotional self-control

   Delaying gratification

   Stifling impulses

4. *Empathy*

   Sensitivity to others' feelings and concerns and taking their perspective

   Appreciating the differences in how people feel about things

5. *Handling relationships or social skills*

   Managing emotions in others

   Social competence

   Social skills

Despite the global interest in his book and the theory of emotional intelligence, it has not been substantiated through rigorous experimental research and the five elements do not correlate with each other.

Trait emotional intelligence model

This model was developed by Konstantinos Vasilis Petrides in 2001 (Petrides, 2010) and encompasses behavioural dispositions and self-perceived abilities. It is measured through self-report. These self-report questionnaires have 15 sub-sections and have been found to correlate well with certain personality tests, particularly the 'big five' (see Chapter 6).

1. Adaptability
2. Assertiveness
3. Emotion expression
4. Emotion management (others)
5. Emotional perception (self and others)
6. Emotion regulation
7. Impulsiveness (low)
8. Relationships
9. Self-esteem
10. Self-motivation
11. Social awareness
12. Stress management
13. Trait empathy
14. Trait happiness
15. Trait optimism (Petrides, 2010)

Petrides recognises emotional intelligence as a personality trait, much as Eysenck did extroversion (see Chapter 6). Trait emotional intelligence has been recognised as integrating the affective aspects of personality which can be seen to be distinct from cognitive ability. The construct has been defined as 'a constellation of emotional self-perceptions and dispositions' (Petrides, 2010). The validity of these self-report emotional intelligence trait tests are still being undertaken and whilst there are some indicators of internal validity and correlation with the big five personality traits, there are problems with establishing correlations with sociability (Siegling et al., 2015).

Ability emotional intelligence

Mayer and Salovey (1997: 23) define emotional intelligence as:

> The capacity to reason about emotions and of emotions to enhance thinking. It includes the abilities to accurately perceive emotions, to access and generate emotions so as to assist thought, to understand emotions and emotional knowledge, and to reflectively regulate emotions so as to promote emotional and intellectual growth.

They refer to emotional intelligence as a 'hot intelligence', an intelligence that is based on things that are of personal or emotional relevance in the person's life and therefore more difficult to measure. They state that emotional intelligence is the ability to:

- Perceive emotion
- Use emotion to facilitate thought
- Understand emotions
- Manage emotion

This ability model of emotional intelligence appears to be very similar to Goleman's mixed model, but Mayer et al. (2004) are exploring the concept from a scientific psychological, rather than the pragmatic, approach of Goleman (see Chapter 5). All three proponents of the different models of emotional intelligence suggest that their theory and its evidence base is valid and credible whilst dismissing the research base of the others.

There are four major ways that most people use to handle an emotional situation:

- *Defensive reaction*: Keep emotions at arm's length by using distraction – i.e. watching an amusing film. May be effective in the short term but in the longer term it may not be of use because the underlying issue has not been addressed.
- *Acknowledge and delay strategy*: May recognise the emotion and the existence of the problem but does not spend time or energy thinking about it. This may be effective in some circumstances.
- *Social convention*: Pay 'lip service' to emotions by expressing awareness of the emotional component of the problem. For example, expressing condolences to a grieving colleague, but then showing no further reference to the emotion.
- *Emotional management*: The most effective way of dealing with emotions. This begins with recognition of the problem (awareness), and then the emotion is used to solve the problem. The emotion makes you ask 'what if' questions to determine possible solutions to the issue. A variety of possible solutions may be considered prior to selecting the plan with the solution, which offers the best way to succeed (Mayer et al., 2004).

 David and Tomo

Case study

David has been working with Tomo for four years, helping Tomo's mother provide the best possible care for him. Tomo is 20 years old and has a degenerative genetic disorder, which has meant that since the time he was 6, with average development both mentally and physically for his age, his abilities started to deteriorate. He now has limited control of his body, which is of average size, and has no verbal language or the ability to swallow. His muscles frequently go into spasm, which causes him pain.

David remains very positive about Tomo's ability to enjoy his life despite the limitations. David says that people think that Tomo has no quality of life due to his pain and inability to

(Continued)

(Continued)

talk and eat but that is not the case. David and Tomo have a close relationship and enjoy a special sort of friendship. Tomo is easily able to communicate his needs and desires to David despite the inability to use words. David says that Tomo is very bright and frequently feels that Tomo manipulates him and gets the better of him.

Tomo likes to hold hands and to receive hugs. Initially, David was a bit uncomfortable with this, given that he is a formal carer, but he now recognises how therapeutic this is for Tomo. Tomo indicates his needs and desire by hand and face gestures and verbal noises. David has to watch the gestures closely to understand, as Tomo's ability to coordinate his movements is limited.

One of the things that David and Tomo enjoy doing together is watching football. Tomo is football crazy and collects all the football clothing, posters and balls. Sadly, when Tomo gets excited watching the football, his body can go tense and lead him into a muscle spasm and pain. David is able to give pain relief to Tomo for this and it does not deter Tomo from enjoying the game.

Activity 8.6 Critical thinking

Read the case study of David and Tomo. Which of these two young men are exhibiting emotional intelligence? How do you recognise this?

There is an outline answer at the end of the chapter.

Whilst emotional intelligence is still a contested concept, it is useful when exploring carers' knowledge and skills related to giving compassionate care. This can be seen when exploring the case study of David and Tomo. David needs to exhibit all the traits and abilities outlined by Goleman, Petrides and Mayer and Salovey, although it is difficult to determine without using an assessment tool.

We can see that David not only needs to be self-aware and able to manage his own emotions, but he also needs to motivate himself to do his best for Tomo. To ensure that what he believes is best is what is best for Tomo, he needs to be empathetic and manage their relationship. This can especially be seen in David's initial reluctance to hold hands and hug Tomo, apparently due to his previous understanding of boundaries in caring relationships. David also appears to be exhibiting all 15 traits established by Petrides, including optimism.

If we consider Mayer et al.'s abilities model, we may also recognise that David is able to perceive his own emotions and Tomo's, and to understand them and manage these emotions. It is unclear whether he is using emotions to facilitate thought but it is highly likely that he is doing this.

It is important to remember that, in a relationship, it may not only be the caregiver who is demonstrating emotional intelligence; therapeutic relationships are rarely one-sided and there is frequently some sort of reciprocity. We can see that Tomo, in the case study, is aware of his own emotional needs and whilst his ability to manage his physiological response to his emotions is limited, David's belief that he might be being manipulated could lead us to understand that Tomo is not only managing his own emotions but those of David as well. This indicates that he is also aware of David's emotions (empathy) and is to some extent managing the relationship. Whilst Tomo cannot verbally express his thoughts and feelings, David is very clear that he expresses these well using other communication techniques.

In the case study, we can see how the concepts described as 'emotional intelligence' are helpful to explore and understand the therapeutic relationship between David and Tomo. Emotional intelligence is said to be important in all areas of human interaction.

According to Goleman, higher emotional intelligence is linked to:

- High work performance
- Physical health
- Mental health
- Good relationships

It is clear to see from the case studies that emotional intelligence, however it is defined, can be a useful asset in caring relationships but Goleman clearly states that it can facilitate increased work performance and physical and mental health and relationships. Mayer et al. (2004), in their review of the studies in the field, offer a more scientific and cautious summing-up of the impact of emotional intelligence. They identify that people's scores on their EI test, the Multifactor Emotional Intelligence Scale (MEIS), do not correlate well with the self-scores used by Petrides and Goleman but do indicate the correlations shown in Table 8.1.

Table 8.1 Emotional intelligence correlations

Poor emotional intelligence scores correlate to:	High emotional intelligence scores correlate to:
Antisocial behaviours such as bullying, violence and tobacco use	General intelligence
	Quality relationships: more liked by the opposite sex
Work performance depending on the profession	Stress management
	Work performance depending on the profession
	Customer satisfaction
	Infant attachment and social competence in the child
	Communicating motivating messages

They go on to point out from limited research that emotional intelligence appears to increase with age, and there are links with brain area activity for parts of the brain associated with emotions and cognition.

Developing emotional intelligence

There is a wealth of books, DVDs and websites offering the opportunity to increase your emotional intelligence to become successful in life. A few studies have been undertaken to explore how emotional intelligence can be developed or improved given that the research indicates it can be useful for a person's social, physical and mental well-being. Despite Mayer et al. (2004) suggesting that EI is a relatively stable trait, they found some evidence to support effort in development. Mayer states that the question 'Can a person increase their emotional intelligence?' is difficult to answer but that to answer the questions 'Can a person develop their emotional understanding?' and 'Can a person increase their emotional and social functioning', the answer is 'Yes'. On closer inspection of the guidance, coaching, mentoring and teaching to increase emotional intelligence, it can be seen that these schemes are focused on knowing oneself (self-awareness), managing one's emotions and understanding emotions and communication skills – all of which have been available for some time.

Self-awareness has been discussed in other areas of this book such as Chapters 6 and 7. Some elements of managing emotions has been explored in Chapter 7 such as mindfulness, DBT and CBT as well as communication skills. The skills used to demonstrate emotional intelligence have been called:

- Reducing stress/stress management/coping strategies (see Chapter 4)
- Emotional awareness/self-awareness and empathy (see Chapter 7)
- Non-verbal communication (see Chapter 7)
- Use of humour and play (see below)
- Positive conflict resolution (see below)

Use of humour and play

Humour and play could also be labelled a coping strategy, along with others such as time out of the situation, emotional release and rationalising (Mann, 2004). In Hunter's (2006) study, she identified that humour and play could also be used to develop rapport and to build relationships. These have obvious links with managing one's own emotions and handling relationships in emotional intelligence. Play is said to release stress and encourage optimism and positive thinking. In guidance for increasing emotional intelligence, humour and play are said to help a person to 'take things in their stride', 'smooth over differences', 'simultaneously relax and energise' and 'help the person be more creative'.

Positive conflict resolution

The literature on conflict is quite diverse but it is identified as being something that occurs in all situations. It is generally seen as a negative phenomenon associated with harassment, bullying and aggression but conflict can also be seen to have positive outcomes. For example, you are caring for an older lady and every time another carer speaks to her she calls her 'my duck'. The older lady was not born in the local area and each time the carer does this, she cringes. You speak to the other carer to explain that you think the older lady would prefer to be called by her name. This creates a moment of conflict between you but the outcome could be that the older lady feels more comfortable.

Positive conflict resolution involves:

- Building trust
- Staying focused on the present

- Choosing your arguments
- Forgiveness
- Disengagement from conflict

If you and the other carer trust each other, you will be able to have this conversation without it causing a major rift and recognise that as with, for example, informing you that you have 'broccoli on your teeth', you are being supportive. Once the conversation has started, if you introduce previous conflicts or criticisms from the past or predictions about the future, the person may become defensive and may choose to defend themselves by being critical or aggressive in response. You therefore need to focus on the present. You also need to decide if this is the right time or the right place to have this conversation; they may be vulnerable for some other reason and it is an accepted colloquialism in the north of England to refer to someone in a friendly manner as 'my duck'. You need to forgive them for not addressing the older lady as she would prefer. Once the conversation has been completed, you need to disengage from it. Perhaps you could do this by offering them a drink as a sign of the end of the conversation, forgiveness and your respect for them.

 Bob

Bob was a 56-year-old man admitted to an acute medical ward with chest pain. He was married with two children at home and worked as an engineer. He was being treated for acute angina and was awaiting an exercise tolerance test. Cardiac enzymes revealed that Bob had had a myocardial infarction (heart attack).

Bob was in good spirits and believed that he just had a bit of chest pain and that this was a sign to slow down as work had been stressful. Bob's pain was under control and he was able to manage his own hygiene needs, but he had limited freedom to mobilise as he was attached to a cardiac monitor and had two intravenous infusions (drips).

Bob was very chatty and I ensured that I spent some time every day with Bob simply chatting as it was often too easy to be task-orientated with patients who were 'self-caring'.

After seven days on the ward, Bob had his exercise test and was told that he would need a triple bypass graft (open heart surgery). Bob's demeanour changed significantly at this point. He previously hadn't thought his condition was particularly serious and he was now facing major surgery. He became very talkative and fidgety, talking about anything other than his condition. Nurses had given him leaflets on heart disease and on cardiac investigations and surgery, but these were unread in his locker.

I talked to Bob and asked him how he was feeling and whether he needed any information and advice, and he stated that he was fine and looking forward to going home after all this was over. I asked if he was worried at all and he suddenly confessed that he was astonished that there was a real problem with his heart. He said he couldn't believe that if he had left things any longer before coming to hospital, things would have been a lot worse. He didn't have a date for his surgery so he was simply waiting on a ward. He had no idea how he was going to recover and whether he could work again. I felt that, although there were a number of issues that were out of Bob's control, there were some things I could do to help and give him back some control.

(Continued)

(Continued)

I asked the cardiac rehab nurse to bring a post-operative patient to see Bob to talk about his recovery and how long it took to get back to work, and it allowed Bob to talk to someone who had been through it. Although the surgery had a high-risk element, seeing someone who had survived and thrived post-op seemed to relieve some of Bob's anxiety.

Once we had a date for his operation, I also took Bob and his wife to the post-operative cardiac ward, and introduced them to some of the nurses and showed them some of the equipment. Although the environment was very high tech and rather intimidating, both Bob and his wife knew what to expect post-op, and appeared to be reassured by meeting the nurses who would be looking after him.

We can see in the case study of Bob that the person responsible for his care had spent time with him and recognised that things were not quite right. We could describe this as 'empathic knowing' with its link to philosophy but we could also explore their behaviour using the emotional intelligence literature.

The carer was aware of their own behaviour (*self-aware*) and was managing this to ensure that Bob was regularly assessed and felt respected. They recognised that there was something wrong (*empathy*) and sought to resolve this *intrapersonal conflict*. They motivated themselves and others (*motivating self and handling relationships*) to resolve the conflict (*positive conflict resolution*) and offered anxiety management strategies (*reducing stress*) such as demystifying the process. It can be seen from this case study that the care practitioner had used their emotional intelligence to support Bob's well-being.

Activity 8.7   Critical thinking

Revisit Activity 8.1: Do you consider yourself to be intelligent? Do you think that it is necessary to be intelligent to be a good caregiver? Has your answer changed?

An outline answer can be found at the end of the chapter.

Chapter summary

This chapter has explored the theoretical journey of intelligence theories to emotional intelligence. The early psychological theories of intelligence of Galton through to Gardner and Sternberg where described, leading on to knowledge and interactions in the social world. Interactions in the social world were considered through group and individual relationships. This culminated in discussing a psychological understanding of emotions and finally an examination and application of theories of emotional intelligence.

Further study

The following website offers a scientific approach to the study of emotional intelligence and is organised by John D. Mayer: www.unh.edu/emotional_intelligence/index.html

Activity outline answers

Activities 8.1 and 8.7   Critical thinking

Do you consider yourself to be intelligent? Do you think that it is necessary to be intelligent in order to be a good caregiver?

Most people in caring roles do not consider themselves intelligent. I frequently hear, 'I'm only a . . .' (carer, support worker, social carer, nurse, etc.). Despite this, all care professionals now are educated to at least graduate level.

After reading about multiple intelligence and emotional intelligence, you will probably now recognise how important intelligence is to your caring role. You should also be able to identify where your intellectual skills are.

Activity 8.2   Example intelligence test questions similar to those used by Binet with children

1. *Question 1*: Horse is to cart what engine is to . . . CAR
2. *Question 2*: Andrew is older than Peter and David is older than Andrew. Who is the youngest? PETER
3. *Question 3*: What comes next in the sequence 13243546? 5
4. *Question 4*: Rearrange the letters *rapsi* to identify the city. PARIS

Activity 8.3   Critical thinking

Explore the 11 factors identified by McGregor by thinking about a group which you have been a part of that have worked well together and one that has not worked well together. Were there any differences in the number of McGregor's factors which you perceived?

Table 8.2   Self-assessment of group functioning

Factor/comment	Worked well	Not worked well
Atmosphere		
Discussion		
Objectives		
Disagreement		
Listening		
Criticism		
Feelings		

(Continued)

(Continued)

Factor/comment	Worked well	Not worked well
Action		
Decisions		
Leadership		
Self-consciousness		
Personality traits, empathy, resource availability, physical environment, the task itself		

Fill in Table 8.2. I have found that in groups where all of these factors occur they are effective, but each individual factor does not indicate success. I have added to the table other factors which I thought might be useful.

Activity 8.4   Critical thinking

Do you think that all loving relationships can be divided into these two categories?

- Passionate love
- Companionate love

I believe I have loving relationships with those I care for, the animals that live with me and my children. I do not think they fit neatly into either passionate or companionate love.

Activity 8.6   Critical thinking

Read the case study of David and Tomo. Which of these two young men are exhibiting emotional intelligence? How do you recognise this?

This is discussed in the text after the case study. It would appear to me that whilst David needs to demonstrate emotional intelligence in his caring role, Tomo is demonstrating emotional intelligence as well.

References

Buckley, T., Sunari, D., Marshall, A., Bartrop, R., McKinley, S. and Tofler, G. (2012) 'Physiological correlates of bereavement and the impact of bereavement interventions', *Dialogues in Clinical NeuroSciences*, 14 (2): 129–39.

Carlson, N.R., Martin, G.N. and Buskist, W. (2004) *Psychology*, 2nd edn. London: Pearson Education.

Dutton, D.C. and Aron, A.P. (1974) 'Some evidence for heightened sexual attraction under conditions of high anxiety', *Journal of Personality & Social Psychology*, 30: 510–517.

Festinger, L., Schachter, S. and Back, K. (1950) *Social Pressures in Informal Groups: A Study of Human Factors in Housing*. Stanford, CA: Stanford University Press.

Freshwater, D. and Stickley, T. (2004) 'The heart of the art: Emotional intelligence in nurse education', *Nursing Inquiry*, 11 (2): 91–8.

Gardner, H. (1983) *Frames of Mind: The Multiple Intelligence*. New York: Basic books.

Goleman, D. (1995) *Emotional Intelligence: Why it Can Matter More than IQ*. New York: Basic Books.

Goodreads Inc. (2015) 'Albert Einstein quotes'. Available at: www.goodreads.com/author/quotes/9810.Albert_Einstein (accessed September 2015).

Hogg, M. and Vaughan, G. (1998) *Social Psychology*, 2nd edn. London: Prentice Hall.

Homans, G.C. (1961) *Social Behavior: Its Elementary Forms*. New York: Harcourt, Brace and World.

Hunter, B. (2006) 'The importance of reciprocity in relationships between community-based midwives and mothers', *Midwifery*, 22 (4): 308–22. Available at: www.sciencedirect.com (accessed September 2015).

Li, J., Vestergaard, M., Cnattingius, S., Gissler, M., Bech, B.H., Obel, C. and Olsen, J. (2014) 'Mortality after parental death in childhood: A nationwide cohort study from three Nordic countries', *PLOS Publications*, 22 July. DOI: 10.1371/journal.pmed.1001679.

Mann, S. (2004) '"People-work": Emotion management, stress and coping', *British Journal of Guidance and Counselling*, 32 (2): 205–21.

Mayer, J.D. and Salovey, P. (1997) What is emotional intelligence?', in P. Salovey and J.D. Mayer (eds), *Emotional Development and Emotional Intelligence*. New York: Basic Books, pp. 3–31.

Mayer, J., Salovey, P. and Caruso, D. (2004) 'Emotional intelligence: Theory, findings, and implications', *Psychological Inquiry*, 15 (3): 197–215.

McGregor, D. (1960) *The Human Side of Enterprise*. New York. McGraw-Hill.

Petrides, K.V. (2010) 'Trait emotional intelligence', *Industrial and Organizational Psychology*, 3: 136–9.

Petrides, K. and Furnham, A. (2001) 'Trait emotional intelligence: Psychometric investigation with reference to established trait taxonomies', *European Journal of Personality*, 15 (6): 425–48.

Salovey, P. and Mayer, J.D. (1989) 'Emotional intelligence', *Imagination, Cognition, and Personality*, 9 (3): 185–211.

Siegling, A.B., Vesely, A.K., Petrides, K.V. and Saklofske, D.H. (2015) 'Incremental validity of the Trait Emotional Intelligence Questionnaire–Short Form (TEIQue–SF)', *Journal of Personality Assessment*, 97 (5): 525–35.

Sternberg, R.J. (1985) *Beyond IQ: A Triarchic Theory of Intelligence*. Cambridge: Cambridge University Press.

Sternberg, R. (2000) *Pathways to Psychology*. London: Harcourt.

Stickley, T. and Freshwater, D. (2002) 'The art of loving and the therapeutic relationship', *Nursing Inquiry*, 3 (4): 250–6.

ThinkExist (2015) 'Socratic quotes'. Available at: http://thinkexist.com/quotation/i_know_that_i_am_intelligent-because_i_know_that/15336.html (accessed September 2015).

Tuckman, B. (1965) 'Developmental sequences in small groups', *Psychological Bulletin*, 63: 384–99.

9 Emotional Labour

Sue Barker

The emotion work that matters is control of the feelings of fear, vulnerability, and desire to be comforted. The ideal self doesn't need much and what it does need it can get for itself. (Hochschild, 2003: 24)

Learning objectives

This chapter's learning objectives are to:

- Describe emotional labour and emotion work
- Identify the development and importance of emotional labour
- Recognise the impact of emotional labour and how coping and resilience can be developed

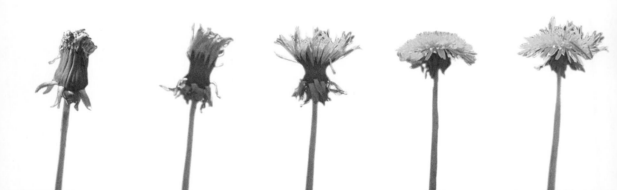

Introduction

When exploring compassionate care it is important to recognise, not only what it looks like when it is provided (see Chapter 4), but also how that care is achieved by the caregiver and the impact it might have on them. This has had various labels over the last few decades, with researchers such as Arlie Hochschild (1979) and Pam Smith (1992) describing the effort to achieve management of emotions as 'emotional labour' in the workplace (aeroplanes and hospitals). Others more recently called working with emotions in maternity care as 'emotion work', such as Hunter (2001). Hochschild (2003), despite being an inspiration for the study of emotional labour, also recognised 'emotion work', but she identified emotional labour as occurring in the workplace and emotion work as occurring in the home environment.

Given this distinction between 'work' and 'labour', we can see that for carers the terms may be used interchangeably because carers provide care in all environments. Regardless of the label, it is important that the carer's efforts are recognised and appreciated to enhance the well-being of both caregiver and recipient (Hochschild, 1983).

To explore emotional labour or work, it is important that we initially consider the psychological understanding of emotions before undertaking a review of how the management of these impact on the care practitioner. As with all the other concepts explored in this book, each psychological perspective has its own theory of emotions.

Activity 9.1   Critical thinking

How would you explain what emotions are to Mr Data, the android in *Star Trek*?

There is an outline answer at the end of the chapter.

Theories of emotion

Charles Darwin (1809–82), accepted as the founder of evolutionary theory, was one of the earliest researchers specifically to explore emotions and, due to the cross-cultural nature of his findings, decided that emotional expression was inherited. Along with Darwin, the psychodynamic approach of Freud and, to some extent, the biopsychological approach of James and Lange, offer an instinctual understanding of emotions. Conversely, behavioural and cognitive approaches, whilst accepting the innate biological ability to learn, would recognise emotions as learned responses to situations or experiences. The social psychological theories of the person, including behavioural and cognitive approaches, can be considered to offer an interactional model of emotion (Barker, 2011).

For psychologists, there is an ongoing debate about the impact of *nature* and *nurture* on the psychological experience of being a person. Biopsychologists and psychodynamic theorists lean towards a 'nature' explanation of psychological phenomena, whereas behaviourists and cognitive psychologists accept 'nurture' as offering more credible explanations. The most recent theorists appear to promote an interactional approach to understanding emotions. These identify that elements of the person's internal make-up, and the environment in which they live, influence their emotional experience and expression.

Emotions involve a **subjective experience**, physiological changes and an associated behavioural change, and different psychological emotional theories are due to the differing emphasis put on each component, from the earliest to most contemporary of these. The early emotions theorists focused on describing and labelling emotions, with Wilhelm Wundt (1832–1920), recognised as the first scientific psychologist, identifying (through introspection) three polar experiences of emotions. These were:

- Pleasantness–unpleasantness
- Acceptance–rejection
- Tension–relaxation

Robert Plutchik (1927–2006) developed Wundt's three poles to eight basic emotions (four pairs), which could come together to provide eight complex emotions.

The four basic bipolar emotions are:

- Joy–sadness
- Acceptance–disgust
- Anger–fear
- Anticipation–surprise

The eight complex emotions are:

- Joy and anticipation = optimism
- Anger and anticipation = aggression
- Anger and disgust = contempt
- Disgust and sadness = remorse
- Sadness and surprise = disappointment
- Surprise and fear = awe
- Fear and acceptance = submission

Wundt's and Plutchik's descriptions are a useful starting point for exploring emotion but they offer little understanding of their genesis and utility. Therefore, what follows is an overview of the major theories.

Darwin's evolutionary theory of emotion

Darwin is known for the development of evolutionary theory through his study of both fauna and flora. His theories all relate to his underlying belief that all living things develop and exist due to adapting the 'best fit' for their environment. Therefore, emotions and emotional expression provide creatures with an adaptation to facilitate the continued existence of the species. Darwin offered three features of emotions:

- They predict behaviour
- The original meaning may be lost as they develop
- The opposite behaviour indicates the opposite emotion

Consider Figure 9.1: most animals bare their teeth by raising their upper lip as a threat in response to fear or anger whereas people raise their lips as a smile which demonstrates friendship and warmth – the emotions of joy and anticipation. This difference can be understood using Darwin's theory, which would suggest that smiling was adaptive for people but its meaning has changed over time.

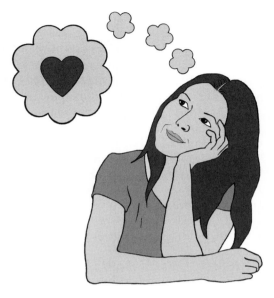

Figure 9.1 Person smiling

James–Lange's theory of emotions

Their theory outlines emotions as an interpretation of physiological changes and behaviour rather than the *precursor* to physiological changes and behaviour. This theory, developed in the nineteenth century, has received significant criticism – particularly from a biological perspective because, for this theory to be justified, there would have to be different physiological changes for each emotion and this has not been found to be the case.

Canon–Bard's theory of emotions

Canon and Bard went on to develop James and Lange's theory early in the twentieth century. They suggested that a perceptual trigger to the emotional response initiated both the physiological changes and the emotional recognition at the same time as these systems were independent of each other.

Schachter's theory of emotions: The cognitive labelling theory

The theories of James and Lange, along with those of Canon and Bard, were further developed by Schachter in the mid-twentieth century. He stated, like James and Lange, that physiological changes occur first but, instead of these being objectively different, physiological arousal was the same – the difference was how these changes were interpreted given the context. The physiological changes were interpreted and labelled using an emotional term such as 'excitement' or 'fear'.

Lazarus's appraisal theory

The idea that emotions involve both physiological and psychological elements has therefore been accepted for some time. Richard Lazarus (1922–2002) identified not only an appraisal theory of emotions but also a *relational* description of them; emotions are related to an experience:

- *Anger*: A response to an offence against 'me or mine'
- *Fear*: A response to facing immediate physical danger

- *Sadness*: A response to loss
- *Disgust*: A response to being close to something or someone unacceptable
- *Happiness*: A response to a positive experience

Lazarus's (1966) model incorporated physiological, psychological and behavioural elements, and with Folkman he developed the cognitive phenomenological interactional model of stress. This is an appraisal model which includes the trigger for arousal, primary appraisal ('Is this positive or negative?'), secondary appraisal ('Do I have the resources to deal with it?'), and physiological, sociological and psychological responses leading to motivation of behaviour (Folkman and Lazarus, 1991). Appraisal theories have continued to develop into the twenty-first century, and there are numerous types available for those exploring this area. They fall into two categories – structural-oriented and process-oriented:

- *Structural appraisal theories* of emotions: Focus is on the content of the appraisal/ what is being appraised
- *Process appraisal theories* of emotions: Focus is on the underlying principles of the appraisal/how it happens

According to Strongman (1996), culture is an underlying linking factor in most theoretical work in the development of understanding emotions. Despite this, he recognises the need to acknowledge that emotions are personal and psychophysiological experiences. Cultural theories of emotions overlap both nature and nurture approaches, with philosophical, historical, anthropological and sociological disciplines all offering a cultural theory of emotions:

> Culture is socially determined and shapes many aspects of our identity, including our beliefs, values and behaviour. It encompasses many factors, including race, ethnicity, religion, gender, sexuality, age, generation, class, life experience [including emotions] and lifestyle. (Thurgood, 2009: 630)

Social or sociological theorists, along with phenomenological and existential philosophers, suggest that, despite the psychophysiological experience of emotion, they are not *reducible*: they should not be reviewed outside of the individual life world or social context and that social process should be considered as well. Sociological theorists have developed an understanding of these social processes, such as power and status (Kemper, 1978), social cohesion (Goffman, 1970), social control (Scheff, 1983), symbolic interaction (Blumer, 1969) and culture (Hochschild, 1983).

Hochschild (1979: 551), a sociologist, undertook research and writing in the area of emotional labour and work or emotional management, and is recognised as *seminal*. She defines emotion as 'bodily co-operation with an image, a thought, a memory – a co-operation of which the individual is aware'. The working definition accepted here for the exploration of emotion work in compassionate care is, therefore, that emotion is the interaction between physiological changes in response to an *embodied experience* prompting behavioural changes.

Emotion management

Hochschild (1983) explored the available theories, including psychological theories, of the person to develop her sociological understanding of emotions. She also considered how psychological theory could enhance her understanding of how a person might manage their emotions. This management of emotions can be seen as twofold: in providing compassionate care, there can be seen to be a need for management of personal emotions as well as the management of the emotions of the person being cared for (consider the case studies in chapter 8 of Mrs Jones, Bob and Dave and Tomo). Hochschild's understanding was particularly influenced by the dramaturgical theory of Goffman (a social psychological theory), to some extent the neo-Freudians (psychodynamic approach) and Lazarus's interactional model (Hochschild, 1979). Hochschild's research has focused mainly on what she called 'emotional labour' or 'emotion management' and the **commercialisation** of this effort. Her research provided a more contemporary and extended application of Goffman's theory of 'playing roles', whilst incorporating some elements of psychodynamic and interactional theory.

Goffman (1959), a behavioural psychologist, suggested that people were always 'playing' a part or role and the person could only be defined by the role they were playing at the time. At different times people are 'acting' or 'playing' different parts and could, therefore, be defined socially as a different person. He developed the concept of 'the art of impression management' (Goffman, 1959), which has been adopted by Hochschild in her understanding of emotion management as part of emotional labour.

Hochschild, whilst accepting the behaviours described in Goffman's theory, does not accept his view of the person. She stipulates that the person has a distinct personal emotional world (they have a unique and ongoing sense of themselves), whereas Goffman only acknowledges the person as the role they are playing. Goffman's (1959) explanation of the behaviour of people, in the public arena, is that they are abiding by the rules of 'the play' to manage others' 'impressions'. He writes of the rules of acting a role; these rules have been adopted and developed by Hochschild. The description of the rules given by Goffman she calls 'surface acting' but she adds an explanation of 'deep acting' in her writing. This is an important issue when we consider the role fulfilled when sharing compassionate care. It has been highlighted by Hunter (2006) that high levels of emotion work or 'deep acting' can lead to 'burnout' and ill-health in the care-provider.

Activity 9.2   Critical thinking

Take a few minutes to think about all the different roles which you undertake throughout the day. How many roles do you take on and how engaged with them are you?

Think about one of the roles in particular, perhaps your caring role. When you are a carer, are you excluding everything else you may do or think? Or do you take features of an underlying consistent self into that caring relationship?

There is an outline answer at the end of the chapter.

Whilst Goffman provided a basis for Hochschild's cultural theory of emotions, others, such as Freud, Darwin and Lazarus, were also influential. Darwin believed that emotions were universal gestures that led to a behaviour or action. For example, the emotion of love, with its associated gestures, leads to copulation; in contrast Freud was concerned with the meaning of emotions and implied emotions were signals. The experience of an emotion for Freud signalled an inner state; for example if the emotion of anxiety was experienced, this might be interpreted as a signal or a sign of impending danger (Hochschild, 1983).

Lazarus's model of emotional experiencing is an interactional model, as it takes into consideration not only the environment and internal physiological responses, but also learned coping strategies (Lazarus, 1966). Goffman, Freud, Lazarus and Hochschild could all offer care practitioners some insight into the emotional experiences of compassionate care. If Goffman's approach is applied to offering emotionally supportive or compassionate care, the care practitioner may be interpreted as playing a role or part with no empathetic or personal emotional experience. Care practitioners could be seen to be following the social or learned rules for the role that they are undertaking.

Activity 9.3   Critical thinking

Think about the education you have received for your caring role.

- Have you been led to use yourself and your emotional experiences to help others?
- Have you been told you need to put your thoughts and feeling on one side?
- Have you been told how to behave and how to feel in your caring role?

An outline answer is given at the end of this chapter.

A Freudian or psychodynamic view of emotional behaviour such as compassionate care might be that it is a signal. This signal could be an indication of the care practitioner's need for kindness, calm and compassion, or it could be a signal of recognising these needs in the other person. For Freud and most other psychologists, all behaviour is enacted for a reason and for most people it is to fulfil personal needs. Indeed, it has been suggested that no one is truly altruistic.

Hochschild's (1983) understanding of emotions and emotional labour, her *interpretive framework*, *deep and surface acting*, *display rules* and *feeling rules* have been influential in the development of an understanding of emotional labour, or emotion management, in all areas of Western society.

Emotional labour/work

Hochschild (1979) identifies that emotional behaviour, as with other cultural behaviour, follows certain rules as indicated by Goffman. She describes these in emotional labour as 'display' rules and 'feeling' rules. Display rules are similar to the social rules identified by Goffman (1959) and have been categorised as 'superficial acting'. These are the rules for the explicit behaviour that a culture or organisation requires of a person in a given situation (read the case study of Lilly – Part 1).

Lilly – Part 1

I was honoured to be asked to go to a Muslim country to do some teaching to the care prac-titioners there. It had been a long journey but I had had a good night's sleep and thought I was prepared for the cultural differences I would find at the institute. My male colleague and I arrived at the institute, we both smiled broadly at the male managers who met us and John shook their hands. I reached out my hand to also shake hands with them as a polite greeting without really thinking about it; it was an automatic reaction. The one manager very gently and reticently shook my hand; the other just appeared confused. Fortunately, I was aware there was a problem and asked if my behaviour was not socially acceptable. They very kindly explained that I was not allowed, in their culture, to touch the men and they were not allowed to touch me. I was also told that it gave the 'wrong' message if I held the gaze of the men, too.

Whilst in this country, one of the managers from my own institution was undertaking a review and when we met in the teaching room he approach me smiling broadly, greeted me verbally and shook my hand. When talking with the students later they had assumed that my manager was a close relative of mine.

In Lilly's case study, there were clear cultural expectations of her behaviour that had social, political and religious underpinnings. These explicit rules are what Goffman called 'social rules' and Hochschild called 'display rules'.

Feeling rules fall into two categories. They are either related to 'superficial acting' or 'deep acting', and these inform the person about how they should feel rather than how they behave. 'Feeling rules', if undertaken through superficial acting, is where the person outwardly behaves as if they hold a certain feeling, but do not feel it inside. Conversely, 'deep acting' is where the person adapts their inner feelings to those that are expected of them within their context. Hochschild (1983) indicates that more organisations are expecting the adoption of feeling rules in their employees alongside explicitly communicated display rules. She informs us that if a person undertakes the feeling rules of an organisation by deep acting, then they may be at risk of losing their sense of self.

Hochschild also goes on to identify that the 'deep acting' feeling rules are not usually explicit and can be difficult to determine. Frequently they need recognising through quite complex, culturally sensitive implied behaviours. Workers are expected not only to know what the cultural display rules are but also to exhibit the associated feeling sin-cerely (deep acting, feeling rules).

Lilly – Part 2

I was enjoying my time teaching the students and they appeared to understand my expla-nations of caring approaches. I had learnt not to touch the men and I was trying, against my training in communication skills, not to hold the men's gaze for too long. I was not sure what amount of time constituted long or short but it was a rule and I was trying to

(Continued)

(Continued)

comply. John was able to express warmth and sincerity using our usual behaviours but I was left wondering how to show enthusiasm, friendliness, acknowledgement, etc. I felt very isolated as not only could I not express my compassion for them; they also were not able to show me their compassion, in a way I could understand. My need for compassion was quite high given that I was in a different culture a long way from home. Gradually, over the weeks, I began to recognise the different meaning in a short smile or look or nod of the head when someone was acknowledging me and when that was done with compassion, warmth and sincerity.

If we revisit Lilly's experiences in Part 2 of the case study, we can identify the problems that can be experienced in understanding the feeling rules and how important that others acting according to feeling rules are for us as people. We can see that the emotional intelligence discussed in Chapter 8 might be able to help people like Lilly to gain the emotional support she needs and her ability to give it to others. Skills in self-awareness, management of personal emotions, empathy and handling relationships are all valuable in her emotional labour.

As established, Hochschild (1983) was particularly interested in the commercialisation (the buying) of feeling rules, particularly 'deep acting' feeling rules and the effort involved in this emotional labour. She found that employers who were paying for their workforce to show compassionate care expected not only certain overt behaviour (display rules) and superficial expression of emotions (surface acting, feeling rules) but also that their staff were sincere and felt the dictated emotion.

This can clearly be seen in the development of therapeutic relationships which all care practitioners will be expected to undertake. The counselling theories of Rogers (1951) and Egan (1977) both expect the counsellor to offer non-judgemental, positive regard for the client, regardless of what the client may have done. This has to be offered congruently: with sincerity. The counsellor in a counselling situation, therefore, has to feel positive regard for the client (deep feeling rule). Although Rogers and Egan were not using Hochschild's interpretative framework, their theoretical stance can be interpreted using it. Hochschild's theory has, though, been applied to care environments by a number of authors, but most significantly by Smith (1992, 2012) and Hunter (2001, 2004, 2005, 2006).

Care professionals' work with emotions

Researchers and writers in care have built on Hochschild's foundational cultural work. There has been a lack of distinction amongst these authors over the definition of the terms 'emotional labour', 'emotion work' and 'emotion management' (Mann, 2004, 2005; Hunter and Deery, 2009). Despite this lack of clarity over definition, there appears to be agreement that, whilst emotional labour is essential, it creates a great deal of work stress for the provider. Smith said that giving emotional labour was, at times, at great cost to caregivers. Nurses appear to accept this cost and provide it is as a 'gift' to those whom they feel require it (Bolton, 2000).

The 'gift' of emotion work

Hochschild (2003) identified that usually gifts are reciprocal, but sometimes a gift is given without expectation of reward. The gift appears to be more than just managing their emotions. Most caregivers believe that they should be caring, loving and kind (feeling rules), and some believe that they should also be calm and detached (feeling rules) (Bolton, 2000). Some, though, have been found to offer something extra that was labelled a 'gift' (Figure 9.2). This 'gift' of emotion work was given to each other in a reciprocal manner (see Lilly, Part 2), but they offered it to the people they were caring for and their families with little or no expectation of reciprocity, hence the term 'gift' (Bolton, 2000).

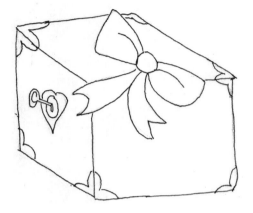

Figure 9.2   The 'gift'

The gift of emotion work is a gift of love; it is something extra, which can be sustained by gratitude and appreciation (Hochschild, 2003). It is culturally determined and so gender, social class and power have an impact on what is expected (both display and feeling rules) and culture is always on the move. Cultural changes within our society expect women and men in the twenty-first century to control their emotions including fear, vulnerability and the desire to be comforted. Despite this, when comfort is offered through emotion management, traditional views still exist. It is then not appreciated and gratitude is frequently not given, as it is not seen as extra or a gift; it is how people expect others, particularly carers, to behave (Bolton, 2000; Hochschild, 2003; John and Parsons, 2006). There is general agreement that emotion work is costly, but this is ameliorated by reciprocity, gratitude and recognition.

It is understood that emotion work, or emotional labour, is anything which has an impact on the carers' emotional state. There is a need to develop caregivers' understanding of emotion in the workplace for the well-being of those they are working with, but also for each other and themselves. The expectation is that this increased understanding will improve their working lives and allow them to meet the needs of themselves and those with whom they work.

The offering of the gift brings anxiety and stress but also brings the greatest potential for job satisfaction (Bolton, 2000). Hochschild wrote that:

> the sharing of gifts is a cultural phenomenon but offering a gift is a sign of love. The sense of genuine giving and receiving is a part of love. So it is through the idea of a gift that we use culture to express love. (2003: 104)

There are a number of writers who accept that compassionate care is a moderated type of love (Campbell, 1984; Freshwater and Stickley, 2004).

Care can be seen as a type of loving interaction which can be expensive and dangerous for caring professions. The dichotomy between professional technical care and emotional compassionate care, in the form of a gift, can also create emotional strain for the caregiver.

Outcomes of offering emotional care

There are three types of emotional outcome identified when there is a need or desire to respond to emotions. These are:

- *Emotional harmony* between behaviour and feelings
- *Emotional dissonance* between behaviour and feelings
- *Emotional deviance* between behaviour and feelings (Mann, 2004)

Emotional harmony is where the emotion portrayed is the one experienced; feeling rules and the personal experience are in harmony. Emotional dissonance occurs when feeling rules and organisational rules dictate a person should behave and feel in a certain way, but this is not how the person would like to behave or how they feel. Emotional deviance occurs when the person is expressing their emotions in a way that they feel is appropriate and is the way they feel, but which does not match the organisational rules or expectations. Both emotional dissonance and deviance could cause distress for the care practitioner but deviance creates problems for the caregiver, organisation and the person receiving care (Barker, 2011).

Emotion work or labour and particularly the 'gift' can be seen as a double-edged sword, in that it may achieve the necessary outcomes, but it may prove too costly for the psychological well-being of the person enacting it. There are a number of physical and psychological conditions that can occur if expectations of a caregiver are too high. These include:

- Immunity and endocrine problems
- Cardiovascular problems
- Stress or anxiety disorders
- Compassion fatigue
- Burnout

A clear link has been demonstrated between emotional labour, stress and 'burnout' (Mann, 2004).

Burnout

'Burnout' can be defined as a state of ill-being where **emotional exhaustion, depersonalisation** and decreased self-efficacy are experienced. Burnout in care environments can lead to health and financial costs in relation to sickness and staff turnover, and may lead to reduced quality of care, failure to recognise individual distress and decreased job satisfaction.

It has been highlighted by Hunter (2006) and Sandall (1997) that high levels of emotional labour and work can lead to 'burnout' and other types of ill-health in the care practitioner. This is particularly the case when there is emotional dissonance or deviance alongside a lack of reciprocity, gratitude or acknowledgement.

Burnout is very similar to compassion fatigue but, whereas compassion fatigue slowly increases over time and the caregiver can still function in their role, the person experiencing burnout may find that they are unable to perform in a caring manner in any environment.

They are likely to develop a loss of idealism or hope that things can get better along with the loss of energy and purpose.

Burnout syndrome can be defined as multidimensional, including:

- Emotional exhaustion, understood as a feeling of exhaustion and failure of the person to give more of their self
- Depersonalisation, in which the person's relationship with patients and colleagues becomes cold, distant and guided by cynicism
- Lack of personal and professional completion, which may manifest itself by a sense of incompetence and inability to respond to requests, or by a sense of omnipotence (Pereira et al., 2011: 314)

Burnout needs to be addressed for the well-being of all involved. It is also important that those more likely to develop burnout are able to identify this and use adaptive coping strategies. Alongside this, managers also need to ensure adequate support for staff where high levels of emotional labour, particularly emotion work, are expected. There is some evidence that clinical supervision (see Chapter 10) and psychological intervention training such as CBT (see Chapter 7) are successful in reducing burnout in care workers. Supportive relationships can help to manage emotional stress, and continuing personal and professional development can reduce burnout (Stewart and Terry, 2014).

A useful and popular model within mental healthcare to explore the risk of developing ill-being such as burnout is the 'stress vulnerability model'.

Stress vulnerability model

The 'stress vulnerability model' was developed by Zubin and Spring in 1977 initially to explain the presentation of schizophrenia, but can be useful for other types of ill-being, too. They identify two type of stress and two types of vulnerability which lie within the person or are experienced through interaction with the world (Table 9.1).

The model suggests that if the person has high vulnerability then low levels of stress are needed for them to develop ill-being, whereas if a person has a low level of vulnerability they can manage higher levels of stress without becoming unwell (see Figure 9.3). The incorporation of an external component to ill-being allows a more optimistic view of the future. People with high levels of vulnerability will need to develop effective adaptive coping strategies but this should offer them the opportunity to maintain well-being. Alongside the individual responsibility, managers need to ensure a supportive environment to maintain well-being. There is a shared responsibility providing both the individual and manager with a sense of control.

Table 9.1 Stress vulnerability

Element of model	Internal to the person	External to the person
Stress	Everyday stress such as negotiating traffic on the way to work	Significant life events such as divorce of parents
Vulnerability	Innate: genes, physiology	Perinatal problems, nutrition, infection, trauma, stimulation

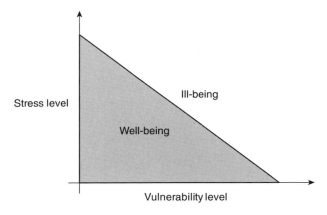

Figure 9.3 Stress vulnerability model (Zubin and Spring, 1977)

A sense of control or the 'locus of control' has been identified as having an impact on people's health-seeking behaviour and sense of well-being.

Rotter (1966) identified that people who believe they have control over their lives have an *internal locus of control* whereas those who believe they have little control over their lives have an *external locus of control*. An internal locus of control can be motivating and lead people to make changes in their lives to improve their well-being. If a person believes that they do not have control over their lives, that things occur due to powerful others or by chance, they are unlikely to attempt to make changes. People who have a high sense of personal control are said to manage stress with less problems. Despite this, if a person identifies that they have a high level of stress which is within their control yet they do not have control, they may experience burnout as they keep driving themselves to address the stressor.

Activity 9.4   Critical thinking

You have just undertaken an examination and have failed. How do you explain this to yourself and what are the implications of your rationalisations?

- Do you think: I did not revise enough; I should have spent more time reading and accessed the tutorial support offered to me
- Do you think: I did not understand what was expected of me because the tutor did not explain adequately
- Do you think: Well, that is just the way it goes. The questions were not ones I could answer well; it will be better next time

An outline answer is available at the end of the chapter.

The stress vulnerability model assists in recognising that stressors need to be managed whether the person has a low or high vulnerability which they have little control over. It is important that those with higher vulnerability develop more robust coping strategies. Whilst an internal locus of control will motivate the person to develop strategies, it is still important that they recognise which stressors need to be endured and which need to be resolved so that the best coping strategies can be adopted.

Coping strategies

The interactional cognitive phenomenological model of Folkman and Lazarus (1991) could be helpful when trying to establish effective ways of dealing with the stress induced by emotional labour or work (Mann, 2004). Coping strategies are usually divided into 'adaptive' and 'maladaptive'. Maladaptive are those which will either maintain the difficult situation or create further ill-being. Some common maladaptive coping strategies are:

- Isolating oneself
- Abusing substances such as alcohol
- Comfort eating
- Risk-taking such as driving your car too fast

Adaptive coping strategies fall into two categories: those which are aimed at resolving the problem (**problem-solving**) and those that support well-being whilst the stressor needs to be endured (**emotion-focused coping**).

Some examples of problem-solving strategies are:

- Cognitive restructuring
- Seeking guidance from others
- Mindfulness

Some emotion-focused strategies could include:

- Time out
- Emotional release, for example watching a funny film or exercising
- Rationalising
- Humour – laughing with others
- Relaxation
- Meditation

As discussed in the section on the gift of emotion work, it was recognised that the stress experienced through giving the gift of emotional labour or emotion work could be ameliorated through reciprocity, gratitude and recognition. It is generally accepted that these are needed from managers and colleagues but there has been a lack of acknowledgement of a role for reciprocal relationships between caregiver and recipient.

Reciprocal relationships

Reciprocal relationship between caregiver and receiver does not mean that the caregiver has expectations of the person, unlike the reciprocal relationships with colleagues and manager. With managers and colleagues, there is the expectation that when the caregiver needs support they will offer it to them just as they have been offered care. The reciprocal relationship between caregiver and receiver can remain 'professional' or 'ethical' whilst still being reciprocal:

> Certain carers, far from expressing 'duty', or 'pay back', saw care as an act of love, being able to provide unconditional care. They could, with shared support from the keyworker, provide the highest level of care and saw this as a true privilege and a highly rewarding experience. (McGhee and Atkinson, 2010: 317)

> For some care workers, the appreciation expressed by older people and their families fostered feelings of accomplishment and achievement. This in turn reaffirmed an individual's capacity as a care-giver, enhancing their self-esteem. Personal growth and development were highlighted as significant benefits of caring for older people. The emotionally laden and intimate nature of care work appeared to help care workers to form a clearer awareness of their own context and the perspective of others. (Walsh and Shutes, 2013: 405)

Reciprocity can be defined as the sharing, giving and taking of a commodity, as opposed to an altruistic giving without expectation of gain. Reciprocal relationships and interactions have been seen as important in the provision of emotion work, earlier in this chapter, when considering the sharing of gifts. It could, therefore, be determined that most relationships and interactions are reciprocal at some level.

In Chapter 7, we explored the therapeutic relationship and the need to engage with those we wish to share care with. To engage with another person and develop rapport, we use phatic communication, but self-disclosure, humour and teasing can also achieve this (Hunter, 2006).

Hunter (2006) identified four key interactional styles in relationships with women – balanced exchange, reverse exchange, rejected exchange and unsustainable exchange:

- *Balanced exchange*: A reciprocal relationship where both are nourished
- *Reverse exchange*: Where the person takes control and the caregiver is controlled
- *Rejected exchange*: Where the caregiver's care is rejected
- *Unsustainable exchange*: Where the expectations are higher than the caregiver can provide

It was only the balanced exchange, or a reciprocal relationship, that offered a rewarding experience; all the others created emotional labour. This is a simplistic model and therapeutic interactions are more complex, but it can provide a method for further exploration of this complex social process.

Whilst coping strategies and reciprocal relationships can support the caregiver, another area of contemporary research in the area of how care practitioners maintain their caregiving without burning out is resilience.

Resilience

The etymology of the word 'resilience' is from the Latin verb *resilire*, meaning to 'leap back' or 'spring back'. When used in psychology, this term describes the ability to recover from negative emotional experiences and flexibly adapt to the requirements of stressful experiences (Hu et al., 2015). Resilience can be seen as the ability to be flexible and adaptable in response to internal or external stressors in a way that maintains the individual's well-being.

There are problems with the definition and research pertaining to resilience as the concept has not been well defined – with its definitions incorporating other ill-defined concepts such as coping. Resilience has also been identified as a category of personality traits and as a process.

Personality traits

The personality traits that are linked to maintaining well-being at times of stress are:

- Positive attitude
- Optimism and sense of humour
- Active coping
- Cognitive flexibility
- Moral compass

Well-being is also identified in those who undertake physical exercise and have social support and good role models (Robertson and Cooper, 2013); they identify four key components of resilience:

- Adaptability
- Confidence
- Social support
- Purposefulness

The above personality traits that have been established for maintenance of well-being are very similar to those identified as underlying the demonstration of resilience. The individual personality traits, which have been linked to resilience, were seen in the same theoretical way in Chapter 8 for emotional intelligence and also correlate well with those for well-being. Resilience appears to include traits of:

- Good self-esteem
- Good planning skills
- Easy temperament
- Mental flexibility

Along with these individual traits, the person demonstrating resilience also has good support networks including their family. The core personality type or collection of traits has been termed 'ego resilience'. People exhibiting this are said to be optimistic and curious and have the mental capacity to conceptualise problems.

Process

As identified above, resilience has also been conceptualised as a process as well as traits held by the individual. A process of resilience has been diagrammatically laid out in Figure 9.4. This demonstrates the factors influencing resilience; the resources available to the person including their personality and social support, their age, and position on the lifespan. Resilience is the motivating force to navigate adversity or disruption, leading to social and psychological outcomes (Davydov et al., 2010).

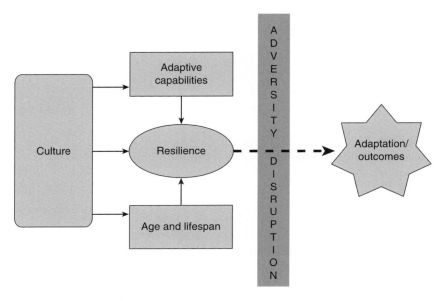

Figure 9.4   Process model of resilience

Resilience as a construct of personality or as a conceptual process is useful in the contemporary exploration of the phenomenon. Whereas emotional intelligence offers an integrated model of personality and ability, the two elements of the earlier theories of resilience have not moved together to provide a dual or mixed theory. Health psychologists recognising the importance of resilience have applied the model associated with their underlying principle of a biopsychosocial model of the person to enhance the acceptance that resilience is not one personality trait but a complex phenomenon.

Case study

 Ciara

I have been supporting a mother and child as part of my role as a support worker with social services based in the local family centre. Both mother and child were considered to be at risk as the mother's boyfriend and the child's father had been observed to be verbally aggressive towards her and the child. The small family had been invited to undertake parenting classes but had refused and had been offered appointments with a paediatrician that they had not attended.

The child was noticed to be lacking in confidence and not following the expected developmental path at nursery. I had therefore been asked to visit the mother at home and support her with organising structured play as part of positive parenting. The young mother appeared to be very grateful for the intervention offered by the centre.

On my first visit I sat with the mother and child (the father was absent); we talked about what they did when the child was not at nursery and I was introduced to the child's favourite toys. The mother seemed anxious to start with but when I started interacting with the child and his toys she became more relaxed and was able to show me some of the games they played such as 'peekaboo'. I felt we were getting on well and that mother and child might be persuaded to do some sessions at the centre rather than me visiting them.

On my second visit, I was expecting the mother to be pleased to see me and the child ready to interact but they both appeared tense and the atmosphere was a little uncomfortable. I am usually a positive, lively person and find it easy to interact with children, and my warmth usually engages adults as well. I quickly became aware that there was someone else in the flat. I said to the child, 'Is your daddy at home?' The mother visibly cringed, so I asked her if this was a bad time for me to visit. She started to mumble and suddenly her boyfriend came round the corner and shouted expletives at me, referring to my interfering in their lives and making them all stressed out. The mother started apologising and the child clung to her. I asked the mother if there was anything she would like me to do and she said, 'No. It's best that you just leave,' so I did.

When I returned to the family centre, I reported what had happened to the team and the social worker said that they would organise a case conference. I was asked to write a statement about what had happened to go into the child's file. The staff at the centre were lovely. They gave me a hot drink and sat me down and discussed with me how I felt. I was a bit tearful and they were very kind about it.

A case conference was duly set up and the mother and father of the child were invited, along with a representative from the nursery, paediatrician, social worker and me. The mother and father attended, both dressed looking smart. At the case conference, I had to share the statement that I had made after the visit. I hated it but I managed to hold myself together and give my statement as well as answer questions about it.

Biopsychosocial model of resilience

The biopsychosocial model of resilience incorporates the major elements included in other psychological health models, in this case harm reduction, protective factors and promotion factors at intrapersonal, interpersonal and societal levels. This biopsychosocial model which underpins health psychology can offer a structure for understanding and exploring resilience (see Table 9.2).

Ciara's experience in her case study can be considered to be frightening, both for her personally but also because she may have been fearful for the mother and child as well. She needed to exhibit emotional intelligence, involving emotional labour including emotion work. Despite her fear for herself, she still remained and checked if she could help the mother and child. The case conference was also an event where she needed to manage her emotions.

We can see that Ciara had personality traits that would enable her resilience such as her positive personality, and her resilience leading her through the process of accessing her resources to manage adversity. The biopsychosocial model as laid out in Table 9.2 offers a structure to explore her resilience (see Table 9.3).

Table 9.2 Biopsychosocial matrix for understanding resilience

Level	Harm reduction	Protective factors	Promotion
Intrapersonal	What elements in the person reduce risk of harm? E.g. personality traits	What elements in the person provide protection? E.g. emotional coping strategies	What elements in the person facilitate promotion of their well-being? E.g. problem-solving coping strategies
Interpersonal	What elements between people reduce risk of harm? E.g. emotional support	What elements between people provide protection? E.g. social support	What elements between people facilitate promotion of their well-being? E.g. role-modelling
Societal	What elements within organisations reduce risk of harm? E.g. policies and legislation	What elements within organisations provide protection? E.g. structures which facilitate social support	What elements within organisations facilitate promotion of their well-being? E.g. personal development reviews

Table 9.3 Case study of Ciara in the grid of Table 9.2

Level	Harm reduction	Protective factors	Promotion
Intrapersonal	What elements in the person reduce risk of harm? Ciara's warm, positive personality traits	What elements within the person provide protection? Her acceptance and appreciation of the support available for her	What elements in the person facilitate promotion of their well-being? Her talking to others at the family centre about what happened
Interpersonal	What elements between people reduce risk of harm? Others showing empathy, care and concern for Ciara	What elements between people provide protection? Ciara was taken to a safe place to express her emotions	What elements between people facilitate promotion of their well-being? Ciara was guided through the processes that she needed to go through for herself and the family
Societal	What elements within organisations reduce risk of harm? The family centre where Ciara is employed will have policies related to a 'duty to care' for their employees and safeguarding legislation for mother and child	What elements within organisations provide protection? The employer will have procedures to ensure that they are addressing the legislation. Ciara did not have formal supervision but she was given the opportunity to talk about the incident. For the mother and child, there was the opportunity through the case conference to assess their support needs	What elements within organisations facilitate promotion of their well-being? Ciara will have annual appraisals and a personal development plan as part of her employment. Through the case conference, plans will be made to address the needs of the family

Resilience, whether regarded as personality traits, a process or a biopsychosocial matrix, actively enhances positive psychological well-being (Davydov et al., 2010). Therefore we need to consider how it can be developed and enhanced to facilitate well-being and reduce burnout.

Developing resilience

Resilience is about maintaining well-being under adversity as well as recovery; its origin lies in both experience and underlying psychological make-up, but it is not a fixed trait and it can be developed (Robertson and Cooper, 2013). There is some evidence to suggest that it can be developed through CBT training workshops, which teach cognitive appraisal and stress management techniques such as defusing catastrophic thinking, dealing with counterproductive beliefs, cognitive problem-solving, developing social support networks and enhanced coping strategies (Stewart and Terry, 2014). Clinical supervision which enhances the development of emotional intelligence could also help caregivers manage emotional stress (ibid.). The strongest evidence to support the propagation of resilience is the development of reflective learning and the improvement of knowledge, skills and attitudes towards those being cared for (ibid.). Kinman and Grant (2011) state that education that enhances interpersonal and intrapersonal emotional competence is likely to encourage resilience, which has the potential to protect the future well-being of both caregivers and receivers alike.

Chapter summary

At the beginning of this chapter, a quote was provided from Hochschild's book. It did not present her point of view but was and is a useful start to explore emotional labour. In her book, she suggested that contemporary culture expects people to look after themselves and to manage their emotions. This does appear to be true for at least part of Western society but there are groups within society that encourage emotional outpouring. Regardless of which view is taken, humans on the whole experience emotions and these at least to some degree need managing. For those who work in service industries such as customer services, health or social care, they are expected to manage not only their own emotions but those of others, too.

This chapter explored what emotional labour and emotion work are: emotional labour is the managing of emotions in the workplace and emotion work the management of emotion in the home environment. Within healthcare, practitioners work in both these areas but social care practitioners mostly provide care in the home environment.

The outcomes of managing emotions for the caregiver were then explored through the research related to burnout. Understanding how to ameliorate and reduce burnout was undertaken using the stress vulnerability model, coping strategies, reciprocal relationships and resilience.

Further study

The American Psychological Society website has information on resilience and how to develop it. You can navigate most of the site and get definitions of psychology, information on what psychologists do, relationships, trauma and other such topics along with their guidance information. You can create an account with them and get access to more information. The following link takes you to the resilience literature but you can also navigate to other sections of their website for this page. See: www.apa.org/helpcenter/road-resilience.aspx

Activity outline answers

Activity 9.1   Critical thinking

How would you explain what emotions are to Mr Data, the android from *Star Trek*?

Mr Data does not experience emotions so it would not be sufficient to explain them in terms of how it feels: he does not feel. Emotions could be explained in behavioural terms ('To achieve this, I express this type of emotion in this way') or physiological terms (the neurological and immunological changes), and there may be some use in explaining them as motivational ('The experience of this emotional label leads me to do these things').

Activity 9.2   Critical thinking

Take a few minutes to think about all the different roles you undertake throughout the day. How many roles do you take on and how engaged with them are you?

Think about one of the roles in particular, perhaps your caring role. When you are a carer, are you excluding everything else you may do or think? Or do you take features of an underlying consistent self into that caring relationship?

I have a large number of roles: I am a mother, psychologist, lecturer, wife, dementia friend champion, external examiner, author, clarinettist, cleaner and farmer, to name but a few.

Many people suggest that there is a consistent underlying experience that is themself (their psyche, their spirit or soul) which they take into all experiences and they cannot ignore it. Certainly most personality theories would suggest this (see Chapter 6). Some people also suggest that they can be completely objective and ignore their personal thoughts and feeling to adopt those of the other person when caring for them. These are questions which I think that as care practitioners we need to keep asking ourselves.

Activity 9.3   Critical thinking

Think about the education you have received in a caring role.

Have you been led to use yourself and your emotional experiences to help others?

Most students I teach say that they have been led to use their own emotional experiences to understand their therapeutic relationships and at times to manage them. Early in their career, they tend to feel uncomfortable with this, especially when we discuss the uniqueness of the person and the need for professional boundaries. It is again something we need to continue to ask ourselves, and crucially if we are sharing our personal experiences, we need to consider the ethics of this.

Have you been told that you need to put your thoughts and feeling on one side?

If you are a care student, regardless of which profession, you will be expected to do this at times. On the whole it can be useful, but to manage our emotional labour we also need times to address our own thoughts and feelings.

Have you been told how to behave and how to feel in your caring role?

If you are a care student, regardless of which profession, you will be have been told how to behave and how not to behave in certain situations. Sometimes, teachers and lecturers tell students how to feel as well but these rules are usually implicit, which make them difficult for students to recognise. If you are given explicit or implicit feelings rules, remember that this takes effort (emotional labour) and you will be wise to develop coping strategies and resilience in order to reduce your risk of burnout.

Activity 9.4   Critical thinking

You have just undertaken an examination and have failed. How do you explain this to yourself and what are the implications of your rationalisations?

> Do you think: I did not revise enough; I should have spent more time reading and accessed the tutorial support offered to me

This demonstrates an internal locus of control and if accurate will lead to putting in more effort and maybe success. If it is inaccurate it could lead to hopelessness and depression.

> Do you think: I did not understand what was expected of me because the tutor did not explain adequately

This is an external locus of control through powerful others. In the short term, this may prove to be protective but if it is accurate you need to problem-solve the situation. However, whether it is accurate or not you still need to seek further understanding to pass the exam.

> Do you think: Well, that is just the way it goes. The questions were not ones I could answer well; it will be better next time

Again, this could be protective in the short term. If accurate, next time you may get different questions and pass; if it is inaccurate you will be at risk of failing again.

References

Barker, S. (2011) *Midwives' Emotional Care of Women becoming Mothers*. Newcastle Upon Tyne: Cambridge Scholars Publishing.

Blumer, H. (1969) *Symbolic Interactionism: Perspective and Method*. Upper Saddle River, NJ: Prentice Hall.

Bolton, S.C. (2000) 'Who cares? Offering emotion work as a "gift" in the nursing labour process', *Journal of Advanced Nursing*, 32 (3): 580–6.

Campbell, A.V. (1984) *Moderated Love: A Theology of Professional Care*. London: SPCK.

Davydov, D.M., Stewart, R., Ritchie, K. and Chaudieu, I. (2010) 'Resilience and mental health', *Clinical Psychology Review*, 30: 479–95.

Egan, G. (1977) *The Skilled Helper*. Monterey, CA: Brooks/Cole.

Folkman, S. and Lazarus, R.S. (1991) 'The concept of coping', in A. Monat and R.S. Lazarus (eds), *Stress and Coping: An Anthology*, 3rd edn. New York: Columbia University Press, pp. 207–27.

Freshwater, D. and Stickley, T. (2004) 'The heart of the art: Emotional intelligence in nurse education', *Nursing Inquiry*, 11 (2): 91–8.

Goffman, E. (1959) *The Presentation of Self in Everyday Life*. London: Penguin Books.

Goffman, E. (1970) *Strategic Interaction*. Oxford: Blackwell.

Hochschild, A.R. (1979) 'Emotion work, feeling rules and social structure', *American Journal of Sociology*, 85 (3): 551–75.

Hochschild, A.R. (1983/2003) *The Managed Heart: Commercialisation of Human Feelings*. London: University of California Press.

Hochschild, A.R. (2003) *The Commercialisation of Intimate Life: Notes from Home and Work*. London: University of California Press.

Hu, T., Zhang, D. and Wang, J. (2015) 'A meta-analysis of the trait resilience and mental health', *Personality and Individual Differences*, 76: 18–27.

Hunter, B. (2001) 'Emotion work in midwifery: A review of current knowledge', *Journal of Advanced Nursing*, 34 (4): 436–44.

Hunter, B. (2004) 'Conflicting ideologies as a source of emotion work in midwifery', *Midwifery*, 20 (3): 261–72.

Hunter, B. (2005) 'Emotion work and boundary maintenance in hospital-based midwifery', *Midwifery*, 21 (3): 253–66.

Hunter, B. (2006) 'The importance of reciprocity in relationships between community-based midwives and mothers', *Midwifery*, 22 (4): 308–22.

Hunter, B. and Deery, R. (2009) *Emotions in Midwifery and Reproduction*. Basingstoke: Palgrave Macmillan.

John, V. and Parsons, E. (2006) 'Shadow work in midwifery: Unseen and unrecognised emotional labour', *British Journal of Midwifery*, 14 (5): 266–71.

Kemper, T. (1978) *A Social Interactional Theory of Emotions*. New York: Wiley.

Kinman, G. and Grant, L. (2011) 'Exploring stress resilience in trainee social workers: The role of emotional and social competencies', *British Journal of Social Work*, 41 (2): 261–75.

Lazarus, R.S. (1966) *Psychological Stress and the Coping Process*. New York: McGraw-Hill.

Mann, S. (2004) '"People-work": Emotion management, stress and coping', *British Journal of Guidance and Counselling*, 32 (2): 205–21.

Mann, S. (2005) 'Emotional labour and stress within mental health nursing', *Journal of Psychiatric and Mental Health Nursing*, 12 (2): 154–62.

McGhee, G. and Atkinson, J. (2010) 'The carer/key worker relationship cycle: A theory of the reciprocal process', *Journal of Psychiatric and Mental Health Nursing*, 17: 312–18.

Pereira, S.M., Fonseca, A.M. and Carvalho, A.S. (2011) 'Burnout in palliative care: A systematic review', *Nursing Ethics*, 18 (3): 317–26.

Robertson, I. and Cooper, C.L. (2013) 'Resilience', *Stress and Health*, 29: 175–6.

Rogers, C.R. (1951) *Client-Centred Therapy*. London: Constable.

Rotter, J. (1966) 'Generalised expectancies for internal versus external control of reinforcement', *Psychological Monographs*, 30 (1): 1–26.

Sandall, J. (1997) 'Midwives' burnout and continuity of care', *British Journal of Midwifery*, 5 (2): 106–11.

Scheff, T.J. (1983) 'Toward integration in the social psychology of emotions', *Annual Review of Sociology*, 9: 333–54.

Smith, P. (1992) *The Emotional Labour of Nursing: Its Impact on Interpersonal Relation, Management and the Educational Environment in Nursing.* Basingstoke: Macmillan.

Smith, P. (2012) *The Emotional Labour of Nursing Revisited: Can Nurses Still Care?* Basingstoke: Palgrave Macmillan.

Stewart, W. and Terry, L. (2014) 'Reducing burnout in nurses and care workers in secure settings', *Nursing Standard*, 28 (3–4): 37–45.

Strongman, K.T. (1996) *The Psychology of Emotions*, 4th edn. *Theories of Emotion in Perspective.* Chichester: John Wiley & Sons.

Thurgood, M. (2009) 'Engaging clients in their care and treatment', in I. Norman and I. Ryrie (eds), *The Art and Science of Mental Health Nursing: A Textbook of Principles and Practice*, 2nd edn. Maidenhead: Open University Press, McGraw-Hill Education, pp. 621–37.

Walsh, K. and Shutes, I. (2013) 'Care relationships, quality of care and migrant workers caring for older people,' *Ageing and Society*, 33 (3): 393–420.

Zubin, J. and Spring, B. (1977) 'Vulnerability: A new view of schizophrenia', *Journal of Abnormal Psychology*, 86: 103–26.

10 Maintaining a Culture of Compassionate Care

Sue Barker and Gemma Stacey-Emile

Embodied relational knowing
Compassionate cultural growing
Each other's needs preferring
Together we grow maturing
Together the gift we're sharing
The gift: loving relational caring

Learning objectives

This chapter's learning objectives are to:

- Identify the key components of a culture of compassionate care
- Explore the role a carer may need to undertake to promote compassionate care
- Evaluate the skills you need to maintain your compassionate care

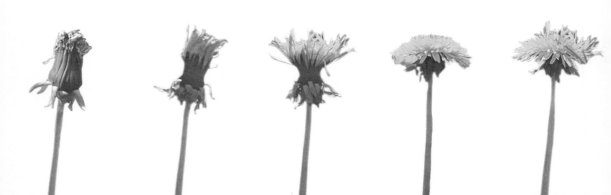

> ## Activity 10.1   Critical thinking
>
> Spend a few minutes to think about what is necessary to maintain a culture of compassionate care.
>
> *Some suggestions are made at the end of the chapter.*

Introduction

Throughout this book, each chapter has considered a topic area to support compassionate care. We believe that to undertake compassionate care, there is a need for a psychological understanding of the person and their social as well as structural world. Chapter 1 offered a basic exploration of what psychology is and the main theoretical categories within it. Chapter 2 used the theoretical categories along with philosophical underpinning to examine human development through the lifespan, and Chapter 3 considered the nature of suffering. Suffering can be seen to underlie the need for compassionate care. Chapter 4 discussed compassionate care, what it is and why it is necessary.

Chapter 5 enabled a deeper understanding of the phenomenon of compassionate care through an exploration of person-centred approaches, their philosophical origins and contemporary issues being scrutinised in this area. Chapter 6 looked at the individual giving compassionate care and how psychological theory could help us understand ourself and others. Chapter 7 unpacked the tools available to us to provide this type of care, and Chapter 8 provided an explanation of the psychological theories supporting the skills that caregivers need. Chapter 9 identified the impact that providing compassionate care may have on the individual and how they could maintain well-being.

This chapter builds on the previous chapters, accepting the philosophies, psychological theories and research already highlighted, which are important to understand and provide compassionate care. Throughout the book, there has been a recognition that compassionate care and those providing it are immersed in the prevailing culture: the **cultural hegemony**. Whilst the contemporary hegemony demands the provision of compassionate care, as has been seen (Chapter 4), it does not always provide the necessary resources (see Chapters 8 and 9). The book, so far, may have developed your understanding and desire to provide this type of care but this chapter is going to consider how this can be sustained. This will initially be done by considering the key components of a compassionate care culture, building on the foundation of this in Chapter 4.

Key components of a culture of compassionate care

Baughan and Smith's (2013) research and model of compassionate care have been discussed in other chapters, especially Chapter 4. They state that the key components of a compassionate care culture are:

- Effective leadership and management
- Positive role-modelling
- Effective and systematic mentorship, preceptorship and supervision

- Ensuring care needs are met
- Legal, ethical, professional guidelines
- Partnerships with all stakeholders

Gilbert (2009) does not offer an explanation of how to maintain a culture of compassion but it could be assumed that his explanation of compassion and compassion therapy offer a **blueprint** for maintaining as well as developing compassionate care, as he states that it is useful for individuals, groups and organisations. He advocates 'warmth' as the underlying principle in compassion, whether towards the self or within organisations. This should therefore be the aim of organisations that wish to promote compassion.

In Chapters 4 and 7, his theory and model were outlined but the essence of his theory of compassion is one of interaction between internal biological changes, external environmental changes and the associated psychological changes. These are experienced through two competing systems: the drive and the **contentment systems**. These lead to a person either embracing an experience or responding with fear. He went on to state that when the person can experience self-compassion through the management of their responses and self-soothing, they can offer compassion to others. Therefore, to maintain a culture of compassion, there is the need for organisations to promote warmth through facilitating self-compassion. To facilitate compassion, the person needs to experience:

- *Non-judgemental positive regard*: This could be seen professionally as treating each other with respect but within professional boundaries, as all organisations need behavioural boundaries
- *Empathy*: Others to understand their perspective
- *Distress tolerance*: Opportunity to develop these skills, such as being slowly introduced to distressing events
- *Care for well-being*: To have the opportunity to care for self and a belief that the organisation will offer them care
- *Sensitivity*: For self and others to recognise current state of being
- *Sympathy*: For self and others to feel for and show care for their feelings

Todres et al.'s (2009) humanising framework, again, whilst not specifically giving an indication of how to maintain a culture of compassion, offers a framework which does not stop as soon as someone has decided compassion has been achieved. Care is dynamic: it is never over and it is part of an ongoing relationship between people and within organisations. Todres et al.'s framework is discussed in detail in Chapters 4 and 5 and can be seen to offer eight poles, from dehumanising actions to humanising behaviours (Table 10.1).

Summary

Gilbert and Todres and colleagues offer an understanding of how people should interact and how organisations should manage people to achieve well-being in all. Baughan and Smith, though, provide a structure which can be explored by staff and managers to maintain a culture of compassion, particularly within care. This will therefore provide some guidance for the rest of the chapter.

Table 10.1 Humanising framework

Humanising	Dehumanising
Insiderness	Objectification
Agency	Passivity
Uniqueness	Homogenisation
Togetherness	Isolation
Sense-making	Loss of meaning
Personal journey	Loss of personal journey
Sense of place	Dislocation
Embodiment	Reductionist body

Manager management

- *Manager*: A person who is responsible for organising a group of staff or organisation; the person who has the responsibility and authority, within an organisation, to organise staff and their tasks
- *Management*: The process of organising staff and/or tasks. The process of controlling people and things

Introduction

It is difficult to know if the culture dictates the management style or whether the management style dictates the culture; certainly to be effective they need to be harmonious. It has also been suggested that the management style is dependent on what is required by the organisation. We can certainly see that large, prosperous institutions have management cultures that reflect what they are trying to achieve. As examples, the Google enterprise with their **bi-generational** team approach to management promotes creativity and opportunity in a rapidly changing marketplace. The implementation of USB's 'united vision and partnership working' and IBM's 'effective manager's approach' of working in collaboration with their clients, who are no longer regarded merely as customers.

Other large organisations such as the NHS have had to make dramatic changes to their management style due to cultural, including political, changes. Initially, the style was more of an **administrative process**, where the managers organised the resources to support the professions, with nurses, doctors and professions allied to medicine managed by their separate professional bodies. The role of the manager in the NHS has now become much more complex, and senior managers are frequently replaced as they are found not to be performing to political and public expectations. The current recommendations are that the NHS develops a strategy more similar to that of IBM – the King's Fund has called this '**distributed management**' (King's Fund, 2011).

The early theories of management style described styles such as **authoritative, laissez-faire** and **authoritarian,** which are useful to consider before examining more complex models. These three approaches have also been used to describe parenting styles.

Martin – Part 1

Martin has just arrived on the ward ready for the night shift. He has changed into his uniform and is on his way to the ward office for a handover. As he walks down the corridor, he looks to his left and sees an elderly female patient reaching for her drink and falling out of bed, hitting her head and cutting it open on the way to the floor.

 ## Martin – Part 2

Martin has just arrived on the ward ready for the night shift. He has changed into his uniform and is on his way to the ward office for a handover. As he walks down the corridor he looks to his left and sees an elderly female patient reaching for her drink; he is struck with how difficult this is and thought that it would be much easier if she was given a different type of bedside cabinet.

Authoritative

Managers who use this style offer guidance and support for the team to achieve the task. This can reduce the creativity of the team but the task will be achieved. Goleman (1995) described the authoritative manager as being an expert in their field of work who is able to clearly articulate a vision and how to achieve this. He identified these managers as having the highest amount of emotional intelligence, therefore as being most productive and having the most satisfied teams. In the case study of Martin, Part 1, this style of management would enable Martin both to achieve the best care environment for the woman without creating conflict in the team and to achieve the best outcome.

Laissez-faire

This is where the manager or parent sits back and waits for the team or child to come up with an idea or attempt an activity. They do not make suggestions or demands. When this style is used productively, the team is given space to think creatively and develop their ideas and ways of working. When this style is not appropriate, whether due to the group or to the needs of the task, the team can feel unsupported and the task is not achieved. Whilst there are situations where this style is effective, it would not be fit for purpose in either of the situations for Martin in the case study.

Authoritarian

This style could also be labelled 'autocratic'. It is where one person (the manager) takes charge of the situation and tells everyone what to do. This can be useful when there is an emergency situation and everyone needs a clear task and everyone needs to work synchronistically to resolve the emergency or crisis as quickly as possible. In the case study, of Martin, Part 1, this would be the best way to ensure the woman received the best care available to her so that her injuries are assessed and dealt with quickly.

These three styles have been developed into six methods of analysing management styles; in Table 10.2 you will find two examples.

Table 10.2 Two methods of analysing managerial style

Example one	Example two
Autocratic: One person dictating	*Directive*: The manager tells everyone what to do and gives clear guidance
Persuasive: The manager encourages the employee to behave in a way that suits the manager's agenda	*Authoritative*: The manager as the expert offers guidance and support
Consultative: The manager finds out what others want but makes the final decision	*Affiliative*: The manager builds relationships with others to motivate and encourage them
Democratic: The manager finds out what everyone wants and decides on the most popular choice	*Participative*: The manager attempts to involve everyone affected by the decision to be involved in making the decision
Chaotic: The manager has no clear strategy for making decisions	*Coaching*: The manager supports, encourages and has faith in each individual and trusts them to achieve goals but can be seen as micro-managing
Laissez-faire: The manager steps back and allows others to make the decisions	*Pace-setting*: The manager encourages others to work at their own pace. They give little guidance, expecting others to know what they are doing and expecting them to perform

Both lists are useful in exploring management styles but, as with any concept compressed into a few categories, it will be limited. Whilst it is believed that these are styles adopted by individual managers, it can also be seen that managers adopt different styles depending on the situation, usually related to the time available to achieve resolution.

Activity 10.2   Critical thinking

Consider the situations in the case study of Martin. What styles of management are likely to be most effective here? (See below for more management styles.)

There is an outline answer at the end of the chapter.

Goleman's (1995) theory of emotional intelligence was explored in Chapter 8 but he also offered six emotional leadership styles. He said that these are styles that can be used by any manager, and an effective manager who has the ability to manage their own as well as others' emotions will use different styles in different situations. His six styles are:

- *Visionary*: Manager tries to lead people towards a shared goal, identifying the goal but not how each individual will get there
- *Coaching*: The manager supports, encourages, has faith in each individual and trusts them to achieve goals, but they can be seen as micro-managing

- *Pace-setting*: The manager encourages others to work at their pace; the manager gives little guidance, expecting others to know what they are doing and expecting them to perform
- *Affiliative*: The manager builds relationships with others to motivate and encourage them
- *Democratic*: The manager finds out what everyone wants and makes the most popular choice
- *Commanding*: Gives clear guidance, supporting and encouraging but expecting obedience

These, Goleman believed, had an emotional impact on employees but these have similarities with other types of manager or leader.

So far we have considered individual management of individual situations but to create and maintain a culture of compassion an organisational response is necessary as well. Effective organisations have senior managers who:

- Are open to new ideas
- Deeply care about employees
- Make employees' development a priority
- Are strong in leading and managing people
- Are strong in strategy selection and implementation (Roe, 2011: 7)

Two large organisations which have been identified as doing well in the contemporary global workplace are General Electric (GE) and the British Army. GE's culture has a key underlying principle of learning to manage its workforce. They aim to identify talent within their organisation and prepare them to perform at their best through a number of developmental approaches such as mentoring and training. This approach appears to primarily use a coaching style of management.

The British Army uses the John Adair action-centred system, which incorporates three interlocking circles called:

- Achieving the task
- Managing the team or group
- Managing individuals

The manager's role is to achieve the task, manage the team and manage the individuals within the team. Considering the management styles already outlined, these managers may be seen as authoritative, pace-setting or coaching. Chapter 8 explored team-building and effectiveness but this chapter is concerned with how these theories, models and research maintain a culture of compassionate care. All the contemporary management theories recognise that management does not occur in a vacuum and that the organisation's culture is important.

The Army used Adair's model to develop five essential elements for managers but they also labelled this role as a leader as well. The five principles which they established that were necessary for managers to motivate soldiers in the Army were:

- Confidence in their capability
- Culture of service and success

- Comradeship
- Complete trust in their leader
- Courage

These might be translated into care environments by using the five principles below, but these remain imperfect:

- Confidence in your caregiving
- Culture of high-quality care
- Comradeship with colleagues, families and client
- Complete trust in the person being cared for
- Courage to do what is in the person's best interests

Activity 10.3   Critical thinking

From your experience of receiving or giving care, what do you think reduces the carer's ability to provide compassionate care?

There is an outline answer at the end of the chapter.

There have been numerous publications exploring what is getting in the way of compassionate care for formal carers. Those identified most by nurses are a lack of time, education and resources. The NHS finds similar reasons as other organisations for not achieving their targets; for the NHS this includes compassionate care. Problems with becoming an effective organisation include:

- Lack of clarity around roles and responsibility for leadership
- Confused organisational objectives
- Lack of organisational data for effective decision-making
- Need for leadership development and talent identification at all levels
- Lack of consistent performance management
- Need to better align individual and organisational success
- Human resources to be focused on the needs of the specific organisation
- A **silo** mentality, restricting partnership working
- A desire to build complexity rather than simplicity
- A blame culture and micro-management – need for more empowerment and trust
- Need for better proactive communication that engages people
- Need for ownership, responsibility, living the values, flexibility, partnership working
- Building an understanding of the wider organisation

Summary

In previous decades, there has been a clear distinction between expectations of managers and leaders. Within healthcare, the manager's role has been more similar to what is now labelled 'administration'. Most theory, research and models of management now overlap with those related to leadership, causing a blurring between the roles. In this section, early theories of management along with effective and ineffective management have been explored. The next section is going to consider leadership.

Leadership

Introduction

A leader is a person who leads. 'Lead' can be a noun or verb but in this sense we are using the term as a verb, which means 'to enable movement, to provide a route to a place or action'. This can clearly be seen to be a different role to that of a manager, which was defined as a person who is responsible for organising a group of staff or organisation. *Leadership has been described as responsibility without authority whereas management has been described as authority without responsibility*. This cynical view-point appears to be justified in the mass media when bank managers are not held to account for great financial losses but nurse leaders are held to account for omissions due to lack of resources.

Within psychology, there are considered to be eight major groups of leadership theories:

- *The 'great' man theories*: Innate theories which suggest people are born to be leaders
- *Trait theories*: Leaders have certain personality types they are born with; this was also a theory of emotional intelligence and resilience
- *Contingency theories*: There is no particular style; some types work in some situations
- *Situational theories*: The leader chooses the best style for the situation
- *Behavioural theories*: From behaviourism people learn how to be leaders and how to respond to situations or environments
- *Participative theories*: These leaders take the role of group mediator and develop the group's way forward
- *Management theories*: A management style of leadership, particularly the **transactional** style
- *Relationship theories*: A relationship style of leadership is the **transformational** style

There are currently many styles of leadership, some of which overlap with management approaches such as the Adair action-centred system. There appears to be a cultural shift towards using the term 'leadership' instead of 'manager', perhaps again in response to media-fuelled stereotypes of the manager as controlling and the leader as motivating and facilitating. Two psychological styles of leadership that provide a distinction as well as a link between leadership and management are the transactional and transformational styles of leadership.

Transactional

This theory of leadership was first described by sociologist Max Weber and further explored by Bernard M. Bass (1985) in the early 1980s. 'Transactional leadership', also known as 'managerial leadership', is part of the management theories of leadership. This implies that there are lots of types of leader with different theoretical underpinning but only one of these is managerial: the transactional style of leadership. This type of leader performs the role of supervising and organising to gain group performance. Leaders who implement this style focus on specific tasks and use rewards and punishments as motivation (Table 10.3).

Table 10.3 Comparison of transactional and transformational leadership styles developed from Bass (1985)

Transactional	Transformational
People perform at their best when guidance is definite and clear	Has integrity
	Sets clear goals
Rewards and punishments are motivational	Has high expectations
Obeying the instructions of the leader is the primary goal	Encourages others
People need to be carefully monitored	Provides support and recognition
	Raises the emotions of people
	Gets people to look beyond their self-interest
	Inspires people to reach for the improbable

Transformational

The 'transformational leadership' style was developed within relational leadership theories. It has similarities with affiliative, pace-setting and participative management styles. Bass (1985) developed the concept of transformational leadership, identifying that this kind of leader attempts to engage the person's internal motivators, appealing to their moral and ethical values.

More than 25 years after Bass's book, transformational leadership is often argued to be the most important idea in business and care leadership. Many students when exploring leadership styles identify this one as being the one they will aim for in future practice. It is a relational and values-based approach. Instead of depending on external motivators used in behaviourism, as with the transactional style, these leaders attempt to engage internal motivators appealing to the person's moral and ethical values – it is more humanistic.

There has recently been a focus on the development of leaders in care services to develop and maintain high-quality care. This has been undertaken in both health and social care services. A leadership framework was developed within the NHS but more recently a framework was also developed in social care by the Department of Health.

The National Skills Academy Leadership Qualities Framework (DH, 2012)

This skills framework for social care has seven sections and each section has a number of principles with associated skills identified. These skills were developed and organised for all areas and leadership levels within social care.

Demonstrating personal qualities

- Self-awareness – leaders must be willing to examine their own values, principles and assumptions, whilst also learning from their experiences
- Management of self-performing personal role effectively, whilst taking account of the needs and priorities of others
- Continual personal development through a combination of formal professional development, personal experience and feedback from others
- Acting with integrity; behaving in an open, honest and ethical manner. Of equal importance is a willingness to take appropriate action when ethics are breached by others

Alongside the personal qualities outlined here, the skills framework expects a leader to work well with others, manage services, improve services and set the direction of growth. Senior leaders are expected to create the vision for the service and deliver the organisational strategy.

Summary

This section has explored leadership. More recently, transformational leadership along with associated emotional intelligence have been encouraged within care services along with dispersed and distributed leadership (NHS, 2008). There has been a promotion of leadership skills within health and social care as it has been felt that these are the skills required to provide high-quality person-centred care. The National Skills Framework (DH, 2012) has been developed to support staff to achieve this. This has led to the establishment of values-led, thoughtful, collaborative leadership. Gilbert (2005) states that a collaborative or partnership leader needs integrity, honesty, approachability, courage and resilience. He writes that these leaders are mature individuals with a strong sense of self which is not diminished by working closely with others.

Partnership and collaborative working

Introduction

Partnership working is another ill-defined concept without a single, unambiguous definition. It has been used interchangeably with:

- Sharing
- Cooperation
- Collaboration
- Teamwork
- Joint practice
- Interdisciplinary partnership working
- Multidisciplinary working
- Participation

Whilst this is generally accepted, Glazer et al. (2008: 4) state that: 'It is our contention that collaboration and partnership are two distinct concepts with collaboration being one component of a true partnership.' They identify that 'partnership' has a formal legislative definition whereas collaboration does not. 'Collaboration' is identified in dictionaries as an intellectual endeavour and can be considered informal, whereas

partnership has legal ramifications – in law it is defined as a contractual undertaking between two or more people. Partners can be held to account legally for each other's activities. It can be seen that, given the legislation for partnerships to be effective, they are dependent on each party gaining the respect and trust of the other.

Gardner (2005) recognises collaboration as both a 'process' (a series of events) and an **outcome** (a synthesis of different perspectives) and goes on to offer ways in which collaboration can be achieved. She identifies that to effectively develop collaboration, the individual needs to:

- Know themselves – to be self-aware
- Learn to value and manage diversity
- Develop constructive conflict resolution skills
- Use their power to create win-win situations
- Master interpersonal and process skills
- Recognise that collaboration is a journey
- Identify leverage in all multidisciplinary forums
- Appreciate that collaboration can occur spontaneously
- Balance autonomy and unity in collaborative relationships
- Remember that collaboration is not required for all decisions

Partnership working and collaboration in care services

Partnership working, particularly collaborative partnership, is working together in a contractual way through intellectual endeavour (relationally both formal and informal). Collaborative partnerships with clients or service users and between health and social care have been dictated by government for some time and it is enshrined in the NHS Five Year Forward View (2014), Together for Health: A Five Year Vision for the NHS in Wales (Welsh Assembly Government, 2011), the Patient's Rights Act in Scotland (Scottish Government, 2011), Transforming your Care (Northern Ireland HSCB, 2011) and other governmental documents. Within care, the services are obliged to work together to ensure the well-being of those using the services and to work in partnership with them.

This need for partnerships between health and social care professionals within geographical communities is becoming increasingly important with the rapidly changing healthcare needs, trends and treatments. Three essential elements have been associated with successful collaborative partnerships: **networking**, **leadership**, and **vision** (Boswell and Cannon, 2005).

There has been an attempt to achieve this through a number of approaches, the most prevalent of which is the 'multidisciplinary team' (MDT); but other terms such as 'interprofessional working', 'multi-professional working', 'multi-agency working', 'team working' and others have been used. Read the case study of Joseph in which this approach is used.

 Joseph

Joseph had problems with his mental health and had been referred to both psychiatric services and substance misuse services by his GP, so I was known to Joseph as a substance misuse worker.

Case study

(Continued)

(Continued)

Joseph was admitted to an acute psychiatric ward via the crisis team out-of-hours service following concerns for his safety. He was actively suicidal and displaying bizarre thoughts to his family which led to them calling the police. He was extremely hostile to them, which was completely out of character for him; he was also demolishing the family home and not making sense to them. When this incident happened, he was placed under Section 136 of the Mental Health Act (1983/2007) by the police as he was considered to be mentally ill, a risk to himself and his parents, but refusing admission to hospital. This section only lasts 72 hours and when it expired he was subsequently placed under Section 2 of the Act for further assessment.

Joseph's care needs were considered at a multidisciplinary team (MDT) meeting which took place on the acute psychiatric ward. As part of the substance misuse services I was invited. On arriving at the ward, we were greeted by the ward manager, who took us to the meeting room; when we arrived there were others already in there. We took our seat and then the consultant psychiatrist who was chairing the meeting introduced herself, the patient and his mother, the staff nurse, occupational therapist, junior doctor and the ward clerk who was taking minutes. We were all offered drinks and the atmosphere appeared relaxed and informal. The consultant took the lead, asking Joseph how he was feeling; he responded hesitantly saying that he felt safer there than at home, but he appeared quite guarded and had limited eye contact with anyone around the table. The consultant asked whether he understood that he was under Section 2 of the Mental Health Act and that he had a right to appeal against this if he would like. Joseph said he didn't mind and had no intentions of leaving the ward.

Each member of the group offered their feedback from their assessment to Joseph and the team, which appeared positive. The feedback was succinct and Joseph appeared to know what was being said by nodding and agreeing with the plans offered. His mother became tearful, saying that she doesn't recognise her son and that this is not him, and asking what had happened to him, and she started crying and sobbing. The staff nurse suggested that they left to go and get a drink; she left the meeting with the mother. The discussions continued without them; Joseph clearly felt sorry for his mother but said that she makes him anxious, too, and that he doesn't feel able to tell her how he feels as he is worried she will not understand.

Within 10 minutes, the mother returned calmer and we recapped for her what the plan was – for Joseph to remain in hospital, for therapy to commence and for Joseph to start some medication which will be reviewed daily.

Overall, this meeting was well managed: the staff attending clearly all knew Joseph, had completed their assessments and they offered a joint and inclusive approach which was not judgemental. Clinical terminology that could have been used was not and the mother was provided with emotional support in a dignified and compassionate way.

Summary

Partnership and collaborative working are expected within contemporary care services as they are recognised as essential for high-quality care delivery. This is legislated for but the government also provides clear guidance on how this can be achieved through effective leadership.

Legal, ethical, professional guidelines

Introduction

As identified by Baughan and Smith, all compassionate care cultures need to comply with the legal, ethical and professional legislation and guidelines.

Professional

Each health or social care professional will have their own code of conduct or similar guidance provided by their registering professional body within the UK:

Nursing Midwifery Council

- Nurses
- Health visitors
- Midwives

General Medical Council

- Doctors

College of Optometrists

- Optometrists

The *Health Care Professions Council* register the following professions but all of them have a specific professional body which also offers guidance:

- Occupational therapists
- Psychologists
- Physiotherapists
- Social workers
- Operating department assistants/practitioners
- Paramedics/emergency care practitioners
- Chiropodists/podiatrists
- Dieticians
- Hearing-aid dispensers
- Radiographers
- Speech and language therapists

Ethical

Whilst there are some differences according to the differing roles, there are ethical and legal principles which underpin all care professions:

- **Fidelity**: Honouring the trust placed in the practitioner
- **Autonomy**: Respect for the person's right to be self-governing
- **Beneficence**: A commitment to promoting the person's well-being
- **Non-maleficence**: A commitment to avoiding harm to the person
- **Justice**: The fair care provision for all people
- Self-respect: Fostering the practitioner's self-knowledge and care for self

Legal

All laws apply to caregivers in the same as any other person in the land, but there are certain laws that have specific importance for care practices. These include:

- Confidentiality laws such as the Data Protection Act (UK Government, 1998)
- Consent laws such as the Mental Capacity Act (UK Government, 2009)
- Administration and storage of drugs such as the Medicines Act (UK Government, 1968)
- Mental Health Act (UK Government, 1983/2007)
- Health and Social Care Act (2012), Care Act (2013)

To provide and maintain a culture of compassion, it is imperative that people are cared for according to legalisation but also to clearly stated ethical principles. Whilst compassionate care involves emotions and the use of self, it is important that carers do not forget the need to be lawful and not mislead people about what they are able to provide and the boundaries of this.

Summary

All registered care practitioners have clear guidance from their professional bodies on how they should provide care. Care services are also managed through legislation such as the Mental Health, Care and Data Protection Acts of **Parliament**.

So far, we have considered the wider cultural hegemony, management and leadership, the need for partnership and collaboration, and the requirement to work within ethical and legal boundaries. The rest of this chapter will focus more on the individual and their attitudes and behaviours to maintain a culture of compassion in care.

Mentorship, preceptorship, role-modelling and supervision

A 'mentor' is described as an experienced advisor and a 'mentee' as someone who is guided by a mentor. A 'role model' is a person who is admired or highly regarded and whose behaviour is imitated, whereas a **preceptor** is a person who teaches, or supervises, coming from the Latin word meaning 'to teach'. A **supervisor** is described as a person undertaking a collaborative professional relationship. This relationship involves both facilitative and evaluative components with the aim to enhance professional competence and monitor the quality of care to protect the public (APA, 2014). All of these terms are used within care services.

The evidence available does not offer a clear distinction between mentoring, preceptorship, role-modelling and supervision as with other significant concepts in this chapter. Despite this, there could be considered to be a hierarchical differentiation from professional or teaching viewpoints between the terms with role-modelling being at the lowest level. Role-modelling can be provided by any competent practitioner whose practice is exemplary. A mentor could be seen not only to have competent care skills but as someone that can offer guidance as well. This could be further developed to a preceptor role where competent care and guidance are built on to provide education or supervision. Finally, we reach the supervisory role.

Ironically, minimal attention has been given to defining, assessing or evaluating supervisor competence, despite the recognition of its need or to determining requisite training. The supervisor is responsible for ensuring the protection of the public within care

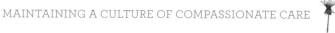

services, which requires supervisor competence. To develop supervisory competence, a practitioner requires appropriate knowledge, skills and attitudes (APA, 2014).

Supervision

Introduction

Supervision has an enormous impact on how staff work. It affects their confidence, motivation and competence. It affects how well they work with colleagues. It affects how they feel about their job and their employer. All of which directly affects the quality of care we offer to the people using our services. (SCIE, 2012: 2)

Within the UK, there are considered to be two types of supervision with differing roles undertaken by supervisors with some differences in style and approach. The principal difference between **management supervision** and clinical supervision is the focus of the conversation. The management supervisor is seeking to achieve the organisational outcomes through the guidance and support of the individual whereas clinical supervision is seeking to guide and support the individual for individual professional development. Whilst this seems to be at odds, they are seeking the same thing as far as care provision is concerned. Both the care service and the professional caregiver are seeking the highest level of care and well-being.

Management supervision

The power relationship is not equal in management supervision as the supervisor usually is senior to the supervisee and therefore has more power. The direction or focus for supervision comes from the organisation's strategy, manager's priorities, campaigns, etc. Any developmental needs have to fit with organisational priorities and budget. The management supervision relationship can be described as performance management. Usually, the supervisee does not have a choice over who their manager is, what skills they bring to the role and how long the relationship will last. Management supervision may sometimes involve disciplinary proceedings. Read the case study of 'Management supervision' in the box.

 ## Management supervision

Case study

During management supervision, there is an expectation to have to hand information that is affecting the productivity of the team. The management supervision that I am accustomed to involves working through a list which reviews and includes performance indicators (quarterly reports about referral numbers/discharges/transfers of care), risk/potential risk (clinical, managerial and financial), human resource issues, collaborated working issues/ networking and future developments.

Management supervision is monthly but if there are risk areas, these will be managed more acutely with regular updates provided in a timely agreed manner either verbally or

(Continued)

(Continued)

written. There is an expectation that information is at hand and that feedback on all the identified areas is available to be discussed and explored in detail if need be. The information discussed is linked to the service development plan and the overarching health board goals.

My manager expected to have all this information in a clearly laid-out plan with achievement dates in place to ensure that tasks were completed in a timely manner and that there was a conclusion if areas needed to be reviewed in detail or developments implemented; this is so that service evaluation could take place when needed.

There is little value in attending management supervision without all the required information as my manager's style of management was quite controlling and autocratic in nature; they had standards that they wanted maintained and did not like these to be deviated from without prior discussion or inclusion.

Due to being rather busy and unable to review the quarterly report prior to management supervision on one occasion, I was unable to review all the discharges. This led to some curt discussion and frustrations as I was unable to answer why we had so little movement in the numbers of discharges for the quarter. I attempted to offer a brief explanation making a clinical judgement but I could not link this clearly to the numbers. This then caused anxiety and questioning and made me doubt myself as their approach was rather direct and accusatory.

Within the management supervision case study, we can see that the supervisee did not have any choice over their supervisor and the style adopted by them, and the power balance was clearly unequal. The supervision was addressing performance and service outcomes. Whilst the case study appears to show a negative experience for the supervisee, the style of the supervisor usually led to structured concise feedback on service achievement and requirements, which are necessary for a service to continue to provide the best care available.

Clinical supervision

Clinical supervision is recommended for all health and social care practitioners, which should be made available by employers to facilitate development of knowledge and skills in the clinical environment. Its aim is to protect and develop the care practitioner as well as supporting the provision of quality care and safety for the person receiving the care interventions.

It is usually provided as a formal process and should be regular and time should be made available for it. The aim is for the supervisee is to gain, maintain and develop their practice through reflection and focused support. Reflection can be facilitated by one or more experienced colleagues or the individual can undertake this privately. In clinical supervision, though, the supervisor should have expertise in facilitation and the sessions should be led by the supervisee's agenda. The process of clinical supervision should continue throughout the caregiver's career (Bond and Holland, 2010: 15).

Clinical supervision can be provided in one-to-one sessions, group sessions or through peer-group supervision. Waskett (2009) developed a model of clinical supervision for nurse and allied health professionals such as occupational therapists. This model was called the 4Ss: structure, skill, support and sustainability. It was developed within Greater Manchester to improve their clinical supervision. It is non-managerial and is solution-focused supervision.

Stage 1: Structure   To include clinical supervision within care services, a clear structure is necessary. This includes senior members of the organisation supporting its inclusion and protected time, along with an agreed policy. The policy will need to include decisions on the logistics such as timescale, resources and documentation along with professional issues such as should it uni-professional or cross-professional boundaries. It also needs to establish ethical boundaries such as confidentiality.

Stage 2: Skills   Once a structure is established, the organisation needs to ensure the supervisors as well as the supervisees have the skills required to undertake clinical supervision. This may include facilitation skills, reflection skills and problem management, and perhaps also some counselling skills such as brief solution-focused communication.

Stage 3: Support   Waskett (2009) highlights that it is essential to provide ongoing support for clinical supervisors. This can be achieved through regular group meetings to share good practice and discuss dilemmas, and these may also provide top-up training. Supervisors should have their own confidential supervision.

Stage 4: Sustainability   Any scheme should plan for sustainability. Initially the supervisors will practise and develop their skills. Supervisees will in time observe and imitate these and develop to become supervisors themselves. The organisation will need to provide some resources to support skills top-ups and ongoing audit/ evaluation.

Waskett's (2009) model can provide a structure and process for developing clinical supervision, regardless of the model used in sessions, whether it is brief solution-focused communication, CBT, a systems approach or a more humanistic approach.

A common model used within clinical supervision in health services is:

- **Normative**: Highlights the importance of professional and organisational standards and the need for competence and accountability
- **Restorative**: A way of supporting workers who are affected by the distress, pain and fragmentation of the client and how they need time to become aware of how this has affected them and to deal with reactions
- **Formative**: Developing the skills, understanding and abilities of the supervisee through reflection (Bond and Holland, 2010)

The characteristics of an effective and ineffective supervisor can be seen in Table 10.4. Using the case study of Ffion you may be able to identify the skills her supervisor was using.

Table 10.4 Comparison of ineffective and effective supervisory styles

Effective supervisors	Ineffective supervisors
Empathetic	Rigid
Supportive	Lacking empathy
Flexible	Unsupportive
Link theory with practice	Indirect and intolerant
Engage in joint problem-solving	Closed
Interpretative	Lack respect for differences
Respectful	Lacking in praise and encouragement
Knowledgeable	Judgemental; emphasise evaluation, weaknesses and deficiencies

 Ffion

Ffion is a mental health nurse with over 20 years' experience. We meet on a 4–6 weekly basis for clinical supervision. Each year, we sign a contract and records are kept for each supervision meeting agreeing the date and time of the next session. We meet for an hour and a half but this can be negotiated depending on clinical issues. Ffion is expected to bring along a caseload list (this contains client information such as care plan review dates, risk assessment information, child protection issues, safeguarding concerns and current medication). During the beginning of the session, Ffion is free to talk about any clinical concerns which are client-related; this could be about how she feels towards a client, for example feeling stuck, frustrated or concerned for their engagement. We explore these concerns looking at alternatives and the context and what we know about the client before formulating an action plan that Ffion is comfortable with. This could include further referrals to other services or a review by the psychiatrist in our team.

During the remainder of the session, we go through all of Ffion's clients, ensuring that she feels competent and confident that she is providing the care needed to fulfil their care plan. We explore treatment options and medication if needed and review engagement and missed appointments.

At the end of the session, there is time for reflective discussion about Ffion's own development, ensuring that she is keeping to her plans of whatever is in her personal development plan for that year. This year, for example, she is completing her CBT training.

During the most recent clinical supervision, Ffion had discussed how she had referred a client to social services due to concerns over child protection. She had recently gone to the core group meeting following the initial assessment and she felt that the social worker was rude and quite negative and making ill-informed judgements about how the family were coping. Following the meeting, the family asked for Ffion to stay behind and they explained how unhappy they were with the meeting, expressing annoyance and frustration with the situation they were now in because of Ffion's referral. They felt that the social worker did not care and that she was rude, and the family wanted to make a complaint but were too scared. Ffion left the family home feeling upset with herself and frustrated at the social worker, wondering why she had not said anything during the meeting.

We discussed this in detail, looking at the situation from different perspectives. Ffion felt frustrated and upset as she had spoken to the family prior to the referral and had gained their consent (although she would have referred without their consent due to the potential risk), and felt that her relationship now was difficult with the family after taking some time to build their trust.

We used clinical supervision to explore Ffion's feelings and to formulate a plan that was comfortable for her. Following supervision, Ffion actioned her plan and managed to build a good relationship with her social work colleague, and the family were able to continue to trust Ffion. Clinical supervision allowed Ffion the time and space to express her feelings in a safe environment whilst exploring her options clearly and constructively.

Activity 10.4   Critical thinking

Read the case study of Ffion. What attributes can you identify the supervisor using?

There is an outline answer at the end of the chapter.

In the case study of Ffion, it was clear that the normative, restorative, formative model was being used to structure clinical supervision and that the supervisor was using their facilitative skills to lead Ffion through the process. The four stages of Waskett's model of development and maintenance of clinical supervision had also been achieved.

Summary

In this section, mentorship, role-modelling, preceptorship and supervision have all been briefly described whilst accepted clear differences in definition are limited. All care practitioners are recommended to undertake regular assessment, development and evaluation of their knowledge and skills to maintain and develop the quality of their care: compassionate care. This can be achieved through these mechanisms. Clinical supervision would appear to be the most attractive to professional carers, given the removal of a power-based relationship as clinical supervision can be undertaken on a peer-to-peer basis.

In the case study of Ffion, reflective practice was undertaken and this is seen to be an underlying principle of clinical supervision. Therefore reflection will be explored in the next section.

Reflection

Introduction

Reflection has been identified as developing from the writing of Dewey (1910) on how we think. Dewey set out five phases of thought:

- Mind leaping to an idea or solution
- Taking the felt sense, the embodied experience, into a concrete describable experience
- Going through a process of thoughts or ideas to check out what fits best

- Mental elaboration of the idea
- Testing the idea

Schön (1983) developed this thinking further to explore reflection-on-action and reflection-in-action. He suggested that practitioners experience each encounter as new, allowing themself to be surprised and puzzled by it, recognising that each encounter is unique. The practitioner then reflects on the phenomenon and their understanding of it. They then experiment either behaviourally or imaginatively to change the situation and develop a new understanding of the phenomenon.

Reflection involves making a choice to learn from an activity, to learn from our experiences. It has been identified as an essential tool to link theory with practice and supporting the development of clinical skills towards becoming a professional practitioner. Reflection can create change and ensure that best practice has been achieved.

Reflection enables us to:

- Identify our learning needs and the ways in which we learn best
- Develop our personal practice
- Develop our professional practice
- Demonstrate competence
- Escape routine practice
- Ensure theory is at the heart of our practice

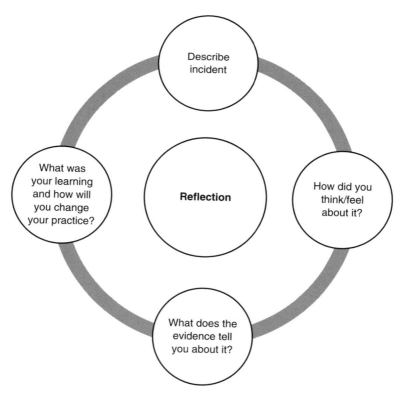

Figure 10.1 Reflective cycle

There are many different models to undertake reflection (Figure 10.1), but all can be cyclical and all involve three elements:

1. An experience
2. A reflective process
3. Action based on the reflection

A common model used within care is the 'what' model developed from Boud et al.'s (1985) triangular representation of learning: returning to the experience, attending to or connecting with the experience, evaluating the experience. Table 10.5 outlines how the 'what' model may be used.

These basic three stages have been developed to facilitate further in-depth learning by adding additional steps such as Gibbs's (1988) and Johns's (2000) models.

Table 10.5 Developed from Howatson-Jones (2013)

Stage of the reflective process	Questions that the person reflecting can ask themselves about the experience
What This is where the reflecting person returns to the experience.This involves a detailed description of the experience	What did I see? Did I do? What was my reaction? What did others do? What did I determine were the key aspects of this situation? What was good/bad about the situation? What were the consequences? What was I trying to achieve?
So what At this stage the person attends to or connects with the experience, making sense of it with the available evidence base	What does this tell me/teach me/imply/mean about me, others, my attitudes? What was going through my mind as I acted? What did I base my actions on? What other knowledge can I bring to the situation? What could/should I have done better? What is my new understanding of the situation? What broader issues arise from the situation?
Now what This is the stage of the reflection where the person evaluates their behaviour based on the previous stage and develops an action plan for their future practice based on this It is the evaluation and action planning stage	What do I need to do in order to enhance my knowledge? What will make things better/improve care/resolve the situation? What are the implications for me/my colleagues/ those I care for? What am I going to do about the situation? What might I do differently next time a similar situation occurs? What information do I need to face a similar situation again?

Gibbs's reflective model (1988)

Gibbs's model develops the ideas set in motion by Dewey, Schön, Boud et al. into a seven-stage model. This incorporated the following stages, but as with all the models it is cyclical – once the process has been completed, the practitioner starts at the beginning again.

Gibbs's stages of reflection:

- *Description*: What I saw/did, what happened
- *Feelings*: A description of how I felt
- *Evaluation*: What went well? What did not go so well?
- *Analysis*: How can I understand this situation given the available information?
- *Conclusion*: What I have learned by undertaking this process
- *Action plan*: How am I going to change my future practice in light of this reflection?

Johns (2000) explored the writing of the previous authors and other philosophers and theorists to develop a way of conceptualising reflection both 'in-action' and 'on-action'. Like Schön, he felt that practitioners could reflect on their practice in processes such as clinical supervision but he also agreed that practitioners could undertake reflection 'in' practice. His book attempts to guide care practitioners to be reflexive in their practice and uses Carper's (1978) ways of knowing in the process (aesthetics, personal, ethics, empirics). Johns (2000: 47) provides a framework for undertaking this, which involves looking in (inside the self) and looking out (looking at external factors).

Looking in:

- Find a space to focus on self
- Pay attention to thought and emotions
- Write down the ones you feel are significant

Looking out:

- Write a description of the situation
- What issues were significant?
- Ways of knowing or understanding the situation
- Aesthetics
- Personal
- Ethics
- Empirics
- Embodied factors (within self)
- Embedded factors (from world)
- Reflexivity (**temporal** knowing)

Summary

Reflection is an important element of clinical supervision and has been highlighted as a means to develop the quality of care. It is easy to see how the processes identified above allow the practitioner to explore what has happened using the available evidence base to develop their practice. Early forms of reflection used a purely logical rational approach such as Dewey and Schön, but in Boud et al.'s and Gibbs's development of this way of learning they incorporated an emotional element. With the writing of Johns, this has been further developed using the developing philosophical psychology related to person-centred care. The last section of this chapter will offer the way forward to maintain a culture of compassionate care through understanding these developments.

Embodied relational understanding

At the beginning of this chapter we shared:

Embodied relational knowing

Compassionate cultural growing

Each other's needs preferring

Together we grow maturing

Together the gift we're sharing

The gift: loving relational caring

We therefore assert that developing *embodied relational knowing* enhances compassionate care. This can be developed and maintained through personal growth and the development of relationships with others. In Chapter 8, emotional intelligence was used as a label generated through empirical knowing and understanding but Johns and others, building on earlier thinking and writing, identify in contemporary philosophical psychology that there are other ways of knowing or understanding.

Carper (1978) offered four ways of knowing (aesthetics, ethics, personal and empirics). Johns's included reflexivity, a temporal way of knowing. Todres explains that all life experiences are temporal and embodied. Embodied knowing is knowing or understanding something through what Gendlin calls a 'felt sense': it is known to the senses but does not arrive at consciousness through any specific sense.

If we bring together the ways of knowing or understanding so far they are all related to the individual: aesthetics, ethics, personal, empirics, reflexivity and embodied. We also need cultural or relational understanding or knowing to share the gift of compassionate care. Embodied relational knowing, a personal understanding through our interactions with others, has been undervalued in our society. Value and status has been given to empirical knowledge to the exclusion of aesthetics, ethics and personal knowing (Galvin and Borbasi, 2012). Todres (2008) developed the characterisation of the kind of knowledge that can encompass knowledge for the head, hand and heart which he called 'embodied relational understanding' (Figure 10.2).

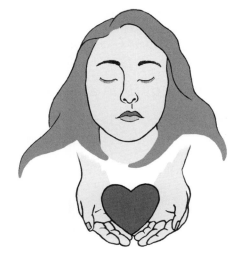

Figure 10.2 Head, hands and heart

Embodied relational understanding refers to a way of knowing that is holistically contextual, a 'form of knowledge that is attentive to the rich and moving flow of individuals' lives in relation to others, is attentive to very specific situations, and to the inner worlds of what it is like for patients to "go through something"' (Galvin and Todres, 2011: 523).

This type of knowing can be enhanced through empathetic understanding (Williams and Stickley, 2010; Galvin and Todres, 2011; Galvin and Borbasi, 2012) and capturing intuition (Rew and Barrow, 2007; Smith, 2009; Traynor et al., 2010). There is a need for leaders, managers, researchers and educators to develop understanding and application of embodied relational knowing if we are to maintain and develop a culture of compassionate care based on the person-centred philosophy. All care practitioners need to use their head, hands and heart to provide the care people need.

Summary

This section has focused on how person-centred and embodied relational knowing may support a culture of compassionate care through valuing and applying the whole range of ways in which people can know or understand themselves and those around them.

Chapter summary

This chapter has attempted to bring together the understanding developed throughout the book to create and maintain a culture of compassionate care through a psychological knowledge base. The chapter started by considering our understanding of the culture of compassionate care and how we could demonstrate that it was effective. It then explored the evidence base for individual behaviours to maintain compassion such as leadership, management and supervision. Finally, it returned to a wider perspective and considered how, through embodied relational knowing, that compassion could be experienced.

Further study

The Social Care Institute for Excellence website offers a wealth of learning material, from video clips to checklists, for all areas of care. It gives clear explanations of relevant legalisation and offers a social as well as personal account of issues. See: www.scie.org.uk/

Activity outline answers

Activity 10.1   Critical thinking

Spend a few minutes to think about what is necessary to maintain a culture of compassionate care.

Baughan and Smith (2013: 175) suggest the following:

- Effective leadership and management
- Positive role-modelling
- Effective and systematic mentorship, preceptorship and supervision

- Ensuring care needs are met
- Legal, ethical, professional guidelines
- Partnerships with all stakeholders

I would suggest that the ability to offer ourselves self-compassion and to truly care for others are the most important factors.

Activity 10.2   Critical thinking

Consider the situations in the case study of Martin. What styles of management are likely to be most effective here?

In situation 1, it is important that the woman's healthcare needs are assessed quickly and that immediate first aid is given; therefore any of the styles that ensure a swift and smooth response will work – such as authoritative, authoritarian, autocratic or commanding.

In situation 2, there is no need for a rapid response, although it does need addressing; therefore a less aggressive approach will be better to manage the situation and maintain good relationships with the team, so a style can be used such as authoritative, democratic, affiliative, participative, coaching or visionary.

Activity 10.3   Critical thinking

From your experience of receiving or giving care, what do you think reduces the carer's ability to provide compassionate care?

I am frequently told that time is the biggest barrier to giving compassionate care. In my experiences of receiving care, this does not appear to be the case as those helping me to cope are also very busy. In the chapter, there is a list of factors that have been identified as a barrier to giving care in a compassionate manner. If you do not agree with these, perhaps you can ask the caregiver whom you know what gets in the way for them.

Activity 10.4   Critical thinking

Read the case study of Ffion. What attributes can you identify which the supervisor is using?

Using the lists in the texts, we can read the following:

Effective supervision

- *Empathetic* – the supervisor appears to understand what Ffion is experiencing
- *Supportive* – the supervisor provides support with problem-solving

(Continued)

(Continued)

- *Flexible* – the supervisor is working with Ffion's agenda despite sticking to the structure of the meeting
- *Link theory to practice* – Ffion is encouraged to consider the evidence base for her responses
- Engage in *joint problem-solving* – Ffion and the supervisor develop an action plan
- *Interpretative* – this is less obvious but the supervisor does appear to guide Ffion through her concerns to demonstrate empathy, which involves some interpretation
- *Respectful* – both Ffion and the supervisor appear to demonstrate respect to each other
- *Knowledgeable* – again this is not obvious but can be implied in the case study

Non-effective supervision

- *Rigid* – some rigidity in applying the process
- *Lacking in praise and encouragement* – there were no explicit descriptions of this

References

American Psychological Association (APA) (2014) *Guidelines for Clinical Supervision in Health Service Psychology*. Available at: http://apa.org/about/policy/guidelines-supervision.pdf (accessed November 2015).

Bass, B.M. (1985) *Leadership and Performance beyond Expectations*. New York: Free Press.

Baughan, J. and Smith, A. (2013) *Compassion, Caring and Communication: Skills for Nursing Practice*, 2nd edn. London: Routledge.

Bond, M. and Holland, S. (2010) *Skills of Clinical Supervision for Nurses: A Practical Guide for Supervisees, Clinical Supervisors and Managers*. Maidenhead: Open University Press.

Boswell, C. and Cannon, S. (2005) 'New horizons for collaborative partnerships', *OJIN: Online Journal of Issues in Nursing*, 10 (1): Manuscript 2.

Boud, D., Keogh, R. and Walker, D. (eds) (1985) *Reflection: Turning Experience into Learning*. London: Kogan.

Carper, B.A. (1978) 'Fundamental patterns of knowing in nursing', *Advances in Nursing Science*, 1 (1): 13–24.

Department of Health (DH) (2012) *National Skills Academy*. Available at: www.nsasocialcare.co.uk/about-us/leadership-qualities-framework (accessed November 2015).

Dewey, J. (1910) *How We Think*. Boston, MA: D.C. Heath & Co. Republished in 1991 by: Amherst, NY: Prometheus Books. Text and page numbers according to the 1991 republication of the 1910 edn.

Galvin, K. and Borbasi, S. (2012) 'Guest editorial: Evidence-based approaches and practices in phenomenology: Evidence and pedagogy', *Indo-Pacific Journal of Phenomenology*, 12 (2): 1–4.

Galvin, K. and Todres, L. (2011) 'Research based empathic knowledge for nursing: A translational strategy for disseminating phenomenological research findings to provide evidence for caring practice', *International Journal of Nursing Studies*, 48: 522–30.

Gardner, D. (2005) 'Ten lessons in collaboration', *OJIN: Online Journal of Issues in Nursing*, 10 (1): Manuscript 1.

Gibbs, G. (1988) *Learning by Doing: A Guide to Teaching and Learning Methods*. Oxford: Further Education Unit, Oxford Polytechnic.

Gilbert, P. (2005) *Leadership: Being Effective and Remaining Human*. Lyme Regis: Russell House Publishing.

Gilbert, P. (2009) 'Introducing compassion-focused therapy', *Advances in Psychiatric Treatment*, 15: 199–208.

Glazer, G., Alexandre, C. and Reid Ponte, P. (2008) 'Legislative: "Partnership or collaboration": Words matter', *OJIN: Online Journal of Issues in Nursing*, 13 (2).

Goleman, D. (1995) *Emotional Intelligence*. New York: Basic Books.

Howatson-Jones, L. (2013) *Reflective Practice in Nursing*, 2nd edn. London: Learning Matters.

Johns, C. (2000) *Becoming a Reflective Practitioner: A Reflective and Holistic Approach to Clinical Nursing, Practice Development and Clinical Supervision*. Oxford: Blackwell.

The King's Fund (2011) *The Future of Leadership and Management in the NHS*. Available at: www.kingsfund.org.uk/publications/future-leadership-and-management-nhs (accessed November 2015).

NHS (2008) *NHS Leadership Qualities Framework*. Available at: www.nhsleadershipqualities. nhs.uk (accessed November 2015).

NHS (2014) *NHS Five Year Forward View*. Available at: www.england.nhs.uk/ourwork/future nhs/nhs-five-year-forward-view-web-version/5yfv-exec-sum/ (accessed November 2015).

Northern Ireland HSCB (2011) *Transforming your Care*. https://www.dhsspsni.gov.uk/topics/ health-policy/transforming-your-care (accessed December 2015).

Patient's Rights (Scotland) Act (2011) www.gov.scot/Topics/Health/Policy/Patients-Rights (accessed December 2015)

Rew, L. and Barrow, E.M. (2007) 'State of the science: Intuition in nursing: A generation of studying the phenomenon', *Advances in Nursing Science*, 30 (1): E15–25.

Roe, C. (2011) *Developing Effective Leadership in the NHS to Maximise the Quality of Patient Care: The Need for Urgent Action*. Available at: www.kingsfund.org.uk/sites/files/kf/developing-effective-leadership-in-nhs-maximise-the-quality-patient-care-chris-roebuck-kings-fund-may-2011.pdf (accessed November 2015).

Schön, D. (1983) *The Reflective Practitioner: How Professionals Think in Action*. London: Temple Smith.

Smith, A. (2009) 'Exploring the legitimacy of intuition as a form of nursing knowledge', *Nursing Standard*, 23 (40): 35–40.

Social Care Institute of Excellence (SCIE) (2012) *Workforce, Care Skills Based Supervision*. Available at: www.scie.org.uk/workforce/careskillsbase/files/skillschecks/23_supervisingstaff. pdf (accessed November 2015).

Todres, L. (2008) 'Being with that: The relevance of embodied understanding for practice', *Qualitative Health Research*, 18 (11): 1566–73.

Todres, L., Galvin, K.T. and Holloway, I. (2009) 'The humanization of healthcare: A value framework for qualitative research', *International Journal of Qualitative Studies on Health and Wellbeing*, 4: 66–77.

Traynor, M., Boland, M. and Buus, N. (2010) 'Autonomy, evidence and intuition: Nurses and decision-making', *Journal of Advanced Nursing*, 66 (7): 1584–91.

UK Government (1968) *Medicines Act*. Available at: www.legislation.gov.uk/ukpga/1968/67/ contents (accessed November 2015).

UK Government (1983/2007) *Mental Health Act for England and Wales*. Available at: www. legislation.gov.uk/ukpga/2007/12/contents (accessed November 2015).

UK Government (1998) *Data Protection Act*. Available at: www.legislation.gov.uk/ukpga/1998/29/ contents (accessed November 2015).

UK Government (2009) *Reference Guide on Consent to Assessment and Treatment*. Available at: www.gov.uk/government/uploads/system/uploads/attachment_data/file/138296/ dh_103653__1_.pdf (accessed November 2015).

Waskett, C. (2009) 'Supervision and coaching', *Nursing Times*, 105 (17): 24–6. Available at: www. supervisionandcoaching.com/pdf/page2/CS Advice Nursing Midwifery Council (UK)(2006).pdf (accessed November 2015).

Welsh Assembly Government (2011) *Together for Health: A Five Year Vision*. Available at: http:// gov.wales/docs/dhss/publications/111101togetheren.pdf (accessed November 2015).

Williams, J. and Stickley, T. (2010) 'Empathy and nurse education', *Nurse Education Today*, 30: 752–55.

Glossary

1-to-1 principle   From Piaget's theory. Each item has one number

Abstraction principle   Counting can be applied to many things

Accommodation   Occurs when new information cannot be assimilated, at which point a new schema needs to be developed

Activities of daily living   A concept developed by Roper et al. in their nursing model. The concept includes all activities as part of daily living: breathing, eating and drinking, mobilising, sleeping, sexuality, working and playing, eliminating, dying

Adaptive   A change that is positive for the organism

Administrative process   A system of organisation applying set rules, programmes and pathways

Adrenalin   A hormone that stimulates an organism into action

Affectionless psychopath   A term coined by John Bowlby. He identified this as an outcome for babies who did not attach to their primary caregiver. It indicates a person who does not experience warm emotions towards others

Affiliation   An association or linking with another person; from the word *filial* meaning 'brother'

Age of Enlightenment   A significant philosophical period running throughout the eighteenth century. The philosophers of the time led a revolution against the power of the state and the Church to determine truth. They identified reason, progress and tolerance as important principles and this led to the increased development of empirical approaches

Altered states of consciousness   Any state of awareness that differs from 'normal' waking consciousness. Consciousness is the awareness and responsiveness to one's surroundings. Altered states of consciousness could include dreaming, hallucinations or intoxication

Animism   Attribution of life to inanimate objects. Everything in the world has purpose; everything is influenced by its mind or spirit, including the sun, the trees and the sea

Apgar score   A measure of the physical condition of a newborn baby; the score is out of 10

Artefact   An object made by a person usually related to a particular culture or time period

Assimilation   The process of incorporating new information into existing schemas

Association   A connection or link between people

Attachment   An enduring emotional relationship, usually between parent and baby

Authoritarian   A person, usually in a leadership or management role, who abides by strict rules and ensures that others abide by these rules, too

Authoritative   A person, usually in a leadership or management role, who offers clear guidance on what is expected and supports people to achieve this

Autonomy   Respect for the person's right to be self-governing

Behaviour matching   Where an individual matches or changes their behaviour to correspond to the behaviour of others. Their behaviour is the same or matches the other person's

Beneficence   Commitment to promoting a person's well-being

Bi-generational   Two generations; two age groups with parent–child spacing

Biological predisposition   The physical body is designed to respond in a certain way which may be due to anatomical or physiological reasons such as genes and hormones

Biopsychosocial   The holistic model used by health psychologists that includes biological, psychological and social functioning to explain health

Blind spots   Aspects of the self of which the individual is unaware

Blueprint   A map, pattern or scheme from which to develop something

Bobo doll experiments   Bandura and his colleagues developed a number of experiments to explore whether through observation a child could learn vicariously. They established that a child would imitate aggressive behaviour if they saw an adult being rewarded for behaving this way

Bonding   A term usually used by ethologists to describe the mother's relationship with her babies

Burnout   A syndrome related to psychological ill health and exhaustion through work

Cardinality principle   The last number said when counting is the amount of items present

Categorisation   Sorting or organising things into groups

Cause and effect   Each time one thing happens, another thing happens because of it; for example, I turn the light switch (cause) and the light comes on (effect)

Celebrate   A response or recognition that something good has happened

Centration   Focusing on the centre, the core of the issue or person

Character/characteristics   Elements that make up the personality

Classical conditioning   Learning by repetition and pairing-association and the law of exercise: the more often it occurs increases the strength of the learning

Classification   Sorting or organising things into a hierarchical order

Client-centred therapy   A counselling approach developed by Carl Rogers

Coding   Identifying something or someone with a symbol such as a number

Cognitive dissonance   Holding two thoughts that are mutually incompatible, which creates psychological stress for the individual

Cognitive restructuring   Reorganising thoughts related to a specific concept

Cognitive shift   Where the established thinking changes

Cohesion   The way in which things come together to form unity, such as a group of people who come together to work effectively

Collaboration/collaborative   Working together, with others

Comfort talk register   Concept developed by Janice Morse and her team – the use of comforting words or sounds

Commercialisation   To offer for sale

Comparative   Identifying the similarity or dissimilarity with something or someone else

Compromised   Where freedom of expression is reduced to facilitate agreement

Concept   An abstract idea or plan

Conditioned/conditioning   Primitive methods for changing behaviour; there are two types: operant and classical. These gain behaviour changes through reinforcement (operant) and association (classical) . It is a type of learning used within behaviourism

Conditions of worth   Refers to valuing things that others think are important to gain positive regard rather than valuing things that facilitate our development towards our potential and gaining unconditional positive regard

Congruent   Being genuine and honest with themselves and with others

Connect   The joining-together of one thing with another

Conscience   An abstract concept related to the mind; the conscience is said to limit immoral behaviour

Conservation   A Piagetian term for the ability to recognise constancy in the natural world

Considered   Thought about

Constant comparative   A continuous process of identifying similarities and differences

Construct   One built idea or concept

Constructivist   A theory of how sense is made of the world – people build their understanding

Content   In narrative approaches to research this is the words within the story. A focus on content could be the meaning of the words or how words are used

Contentment system   A neurological process motivating behaviour which creates a feeling of comfort

Corporeal   Related to the physical body – internal to the physical body

Correlate   Demonstrates a relationship between objects

Correspondent inferences   Psychological theory that offers a process to understand intentions of a given behaviour

Corticosteroids   Steroid hormones produced by the adrenal cortex

Counselling   Talking therapy or treatment

Counterbalancing   Providing evidence or weight for one side of an argument or discussion to achieve balance

Courageous   The ability to behave in the way considered best, despite the experience of fear

Crisis   A moment of significant change

Cultural hegemony   The most influential ideology within a culture

Cultural portrait   A picture of the culture; it could be a picture developed through words

Culture/cultural   The arts, behaviours and beliefs of a particular group of people

Culture-sharing groups   A group of people who have the same cultural identity

Curious   An interest in finding out about things, the world

Defence   An action, possibly psychological, to protect oneself

Deficiency drive   The motivation to maintain or achieve health

Depersonalisation   Where a person's thoughts and feelings do not seem real and they cannot recognise themselves as an individual or their experiences

Deprivation   Where a person has not had access to something that is experienced normally within their culture

Deviant   Behaviour that does not comply with cultural norms

Dialectics   A type of analytical thought for the processing of conflicting objects, messages and ideas

Differentiation   A method of distinguishing between groups or individuals

Dissonance   A psychological feeling of discomfort

Distributed management   A management approach facilitated by working together using systems such as the world wide web to involve the people doing the work in decision-making

Divergent thinking   A creative thought process to consider a number of approaches to problem-solving

Dopaminergic   A nerve system where dopamine is the specific neurotransmitter

Dream interpretation   A technique used in psychoanalysis to understand the person's psychological state

Drive   A motivating force

Drive system   A process that motivates behaviour

Dualism   Two parts that work together for the benefit of the whole

Dynamic   Something that is always in a state of change

Echoing   Repetition of a word, sound or action

Ecological validity   Something that appears to hold true in the everyday/natural world

Ego   In psychodynamic theory, the balancing part of the personality that ensures that individual needs are met in a socially appropriate way

Ego strength   The power, robustness or skill of the ego to meet individual needs

Egocentrism   Assumes that everyone thinks as they do

Electra Part of the psychodynamic theory occurring for girls when the oedipal complex is occurring in boys. It is where girls associate with their mothers when they find that they do not have a penis like their fathers. At this time, they develop sexual fantasies about their fathers

Embodied A person experiences the world through their holistic body. All their senses including their spirituality

Embodied experience Where a person recognises how their body is experiencing the world

Embodied knowing Knowing or understanding something through what Gendlin calls a felt sense; it is known to the senses but does not arrive at consciousness through any specific sense

Emergent properties Things that develop out of the coming-together of other objects

Emic The internal understanding or experience of something

Emotion-focused coping A strategy that can be used to manage stress when the problem causing stress cannot be resolved or removed. It involves techniques which allow the person to continue to stay well despite difficult experiences

Emotional exhaustion Where the person is no longer able to cope with emotional demands on them. They have no emotional energy left to provide an emotional response

Emotion work The management of personal and other emotions in a private place such as home

Emotional labour The management of personal and other emotions in a public place such as hospitals

Empathetic The reaching-out to the feeling, experiences and attitudes of another person

Empathy To demonstrate an understanding of another person's thoughts, feelings or experiences

Empiricism Knowledge or understanding can only be gained through observation and experience

Energy Strength, vitality, power

Epoche The suspension of time and external world influences

Equilibrium Balancing of good and bad, hot and cold, etc. to maintain people's well-being

Eros Freud's life force, the motivating force to sustain life

Essence The core element of a thing

Ethnic   A sub-group within a culture

Ethnohistorical   Cultural development over time

Ethologist   A person who studies animal behaviour

Etic   An objective explanation of something

Etymology   The study of the origins of words

Existential/existentialism   Relating to existence, what it is to exist; philosophical approach stating that every person is the creator of their own destiny: they have free choice

Explicitly   Something that is made clear or obvious

Extinct   Something that no longer exists

Extinguished   Something that is stopped, put out, such as fire

Extroversion   Refers to the extent to which a person engages with other people. An extrovert is said to continuously seek the company of others. The other extreme of this polar trait is 'introversion', which occurs in people who prefer their own company to that of others

Faith   A belief that cannot be proved or disproved by science

Familiarity   Experiencing something or someone frequently

Felt sense   It is known to the senses but does not arrive at consciousness through any specific sense

Fidelity   Honouring the trust placed in the practitioner

Field   In grounded theory it is the place where the information is gathered from

Field notes   Writing undertaken in the place where what is written takes place

Field of forces   The area in which different influences or forces come together to create change

Fight-or-flight response   This is sometimes referred to as the 'fight, flight or freeze response'. It is where an acute stress reaction has been triggered by a feared situation or perception. This trigger sets off a biological reaction called the **hypothalamic–pituitary–adrenal axis (HPA axis)**, and is highlighted in Figure 3.2

Fixated/fixation   Arrested or stopped at a certain point; used in Freud's psychodynamic theory to identify that a person is exhibiting the behaviour of an earlier time as they are fixated on that time and place

Fixed component   An item that does not change

Flexible component   An item that can change

Formal   Adhering to a particular code, strategy, process

Formative   A developmental stage, assisting in the 'formation' of the person

Free association   A technique used in psychodynamic therapy to support understanding and growth. The therapist gives a stream of words and the client needs to give the first word that comes into their head on hearing the therapist's words

Functional changes   The way something works or performs changes

Functionalism   The exploration of how something functions or works

General structure   The bringing-together of the essential features of a phenomenon

Generic   A term used to explain what the norm is; something that is applied to everyone

Genotype   The hereditary information about the person; their biological potential

Genre   A type of story

Gestalt philosophy   A philosophical approach that recognises patterns in perceptions

Grounded   Something that occurs on the basic level; it is part of the basis of something

Growth drive   Growth motives are those at the top of the hierarchy and promote cognitive needs, aesthetic needs and self-actualisation

Habituation   Learning by familiarisation

Halo effect   Where one-word description supports a stereotype such as a warm person and a cold person

Heuristics   'Commonsense' approach to problem-solving; an everyday approach

Hierarchic integration   The coming-together of simple skills to create a complex skill

Hierarchical   Classifying things in order of importance or size

Homeostasis   Derived from the Greek language, *homo* meaning 'same' and *stasis* meaning 'stoppage'. The homeostatic drive refers to the internal body processes which work together to maintain a constant optimal bodily environment

Homogenous   Things that are consistent; one theory is homogenous with another; it has the same meaning

Hormone   A substance that circulates around the body, produced by glands to regulate the body

Hypothalamic–pituitary–adrenal (HPA) axis The fight-or-flight endocrine and neurological system

Hypothalamus A small area of the forebrain beneath the thalamus

Hypothesis An idea to be examined

Hypothetical deductive reasoning This is the basic scientific approach to finding things out. It is the establishing of an idea and then trying to find ways to disprove it

Id Part of the personality as established by Freud. Freud's three parts of the personality are the id, ego and superego. The id is the innate part that is always seeking the fulfilment of its needs and desires

Ideal self What we want ourselves to be; who we would ideally like to be

Idealism Philosophical approach which proposes that all knowledge comes from the senses (sight, sound, touch, smell, etc.)

Identifying Recognising an object's similarities and differences to other things, and giving it a label

Ideology A cultural belief system

Illusion Where an object is misperceived or inaccurately perceived

Imaginative variation A technique used in phenomenology to identify the boundaries of a phenomenon by imagining whether, if the phenomenon looked like 'this', it would still be an example of the phenomenon

Imitation Copying behaviour

Implicitly Where rules or knowledge are accepted but not clearly articulated

Imprinting A term used by ethologists to explain how animals 'bond' with their mothers

Incongruent A psychological experience explained by Rogers whereby the person, not being comfortable with themselves, is not self-aware or genuine. A person may be incongruent with another person, in which case they are not being open, honest and genuine with the other person

Individual variations or constituents Terms used in phenomenology. Phenomenology accepts that there is an essential or core part of any phenomenon but each individual may experience the phenomenon in different ways, and these are 'individual variations' or 'constitutes' of the phenomenon

Inert substance Something that does not easily interact or react with other chemicals, compounds, etc.

Informal   Not adhering to a particular process, guidelines or strategy

Innate   Attributes a person or animal is born with; they are present at birth

Internal working model   A concept developed by John Bowlby to explain babies and children's development and the maintenance of relationships

Inter-professional   Where a number of professionals work together

Intrapersonal, interpersonal and extrapersonal   *Intra-* within the person; *inter-* between people; *extra-* additional to personal

Introspection   A technique for developing understanding whereby the person thinks about their own experiences

Introversion   The opposite end of the extroversion pole in Hans Eysenck's personality traits. Introversion is where the person receives enough internal stimulation and does not therefore need to seek external stimulation from other people

Invalidating environment   A term developed by Marsha Linehan in dialectical behavioural therapy. It suggests that some people grow in an environment that undermines their understanding of their emotional experiences

Irreversibility   A term used by Jean Piaget to explain the thought processes of a pre-operational child. Irreversibility is the inability to retrace a thought pathway backward to the beginning

Justice   Fair care provision for all people

Laissez-faire   A management or leadership style where the manager or leader takes a 'hands-off' approach and gives the team the space to develop their own ways of working

Law of effect   States that when something good happens after an action, the behaviour is likely to be repeated

Leadership   A person who enables movement; to provide a route to a place or action

Leverage   The power and energy to undertake an activity

Libido   Sexual drive, identified by Sigmund Freud as the life-motivating force

Life world   The totality of an individual's experiences

Limbic system   Complex part of the brain near the edge of the cortex that processes instincts and emotions

Locus of control   *Locus* meaning 'place' or 'location'; where control is situated or stems from

Magnetic resonance imaging (MRI)   A technique used to view inside the body, generated by magnets and using computer images

Malignant social psychology A term used by Tom Kitwood to explain a care culture that creates ill-being in a person with dementia

Management The process of organising staff and/or tasks. The process of controlling people and things

Management supervision A meeting with a manager to explore how an employee or employees can achieve organisational goals

Manager The person who has the responsibility and authority within an organisation to organise staff and their tasks

Maturational theory A theory which identifies that organisms grow and change throughout their lifespan

Mentor A person who offers guidance and support

Modelling Where the behaviour of one individual is copied by another

Monotropy The term used by John Bowlby to explain that there is only one way for a baby to grow into a healthy social adult. He says that if the child does not have a consistent relationship with their mother in their early years, they will become deviant or develop psychopathology

Multidisciplinary The coming-together of people with different training

Narcissistic In psychology, this is a personality type whereby the person is only concerned with themselves

Networking Connecting with others to share thoughts, ideas, etc.

Neuroendocrine cells Nerve cells that infiltrate the endocrine glands

Neuroticism One of the polar traits of personality identified by Eysenck. It relates to how much a person worries or is anxious

Neurotransmitter A chemical messenger that carries messages across the nerve synapse or neuromuscular junction

Non-judgemental positive regard Identified by Rogers as a necessary requirement for a sense of well-being to achieve self-actualisation. It is the provision of warmth and encouragement without conditions

Non-maleficence A commitment to avoiding harm to the person

Normative A normalising approach, bringing a conversation back to the everyday

Number concepts From Piaget's theory which indicates that the preoperational child does not have the concept of numbers. They do not understand what numerical symbols mean

Object permanence   From Piaget's theory. He identified that the baby does not have a sense of object permanence, so if the baby cannot see an object it does not exist

Oedipal   From Freud's psychosexual developmental psychodynamic theory. This is the phase which boys go through at about 4 years of age. The boy becomes sexually attracted to his mother but fears that his father will castrate him if he responds to this, so the boy tries to become similar to his father

Ontology   The study of the meaning of living; of being

Operant conditioning   Learning through reinforcement and punishment (reward)

Order-irrelevance principle   From Piaget's theory. It does not matter where you start: you still have the same number of the given items

Organismic   By, with, in or from the organism

Organismic valuing process (OVP)   From Rogers' theory. This occurs when people value things that support their reaching their potential

Orthogenetic principle   Where *ortho* means 'direction', so the principle is that genes ('genetic') provide the direction ('ortho') for development

Outcome   A synthesis of different perspectives

Paradigm   A model or pattern that is typical of a certain style

Paraphrasing   A communication technique whereby the listener rephrases what the speaker has said and feeds this back to them

Parapraxis   The common term is 'Freudian slip'. It is where a person says something, usually of a sexual nature, that discloses their true thoughts or feelings

Parliament   In the UK, it consists of the Sovereign, the House of Lords and the House of Commons. These together provide the legislator for the country

Participant observers   This is a research technique whereby the person collecting the data is also part of the situation being observed

Partnership   In law, this is defined as a contractual undertaking between two or more people

Perceptual constancy   Where an object is seen as the same size, shape, etc., despite changing the stimulus reaching the senses

Perceptual field   The scope of the perception, for example the hearing range, etc.

Perceptual hypothesis   An idea we have about the world based on previous perceptions which we then verify through the senses

Perceptual world   Understanding of the world based on information from the senses

Person-centred care   There is no single precise definition of this term but it generally involves respect, dignity and recognising individual needs and desires

Personhood   Kitwood highlighted the importance of personhood, identifying it as something that is bestowed on an individual by others. It is the recognition of the individual as a person with feelings, thoughts and rights

Perspectives   Different ways of viewing the same phenomenon

Phenomenological field   This is the individual's subjective experiences of the world, which is always changing. The person's world, the phenomenological field, is their perception of their experiences. Their perceptual field provides the person with a sense of reality; it is their personal reality

Phenotype   The observable and measurable features of an individual; the composite of natural (genes, biology, etc.) and environmental (food, relationships, etc.) influences on the person

Pituitary gland   A pea-sized gland that hangs beneath the hypothalamus in the brain. It plays a significant role in growth, development and functioning

Polar   Extreme opposing characteristics at each end of a personality trait continuum

Positive person work   Developed by Kitwood as a way to develop a culture facilitating well-being

Positive regard   A warm way of perceiving and responding to others

Positivism/positivist philosophy   A philosophy to understand people which only accepts evidence that is observable and measurable

Potential   What someone is capable of achieving

Power base   Where the power or control is located

Preceptor   A teacher or instructor

Preconscious   Elements of the mind that can be retrieved but do not appear automatically to consciousness

Privation   A term used by Bowlby to refer to a baby or child not receiving a warm, loving relationship

Problem solving coping   Where the person uses a technique which resolves the problem or makes it go away and they therefore no longer need to cope with it

Process   A series of events

Progressive relaxation   A step-by-step method of achieving relaxation, the amelioration of tension in the body

Proximity   Nearness; closeness in time, space or relationship

Psychoanalysis   A psychological method for exploring the unconscious mind so that painful, repressed experiences can be resolved

Psychoticism   A personality trait identified by Eysenck referring to how well a person 'fits' in with their culture

Punishment   An unpleasant experience used to deter certain behaviour

Qualitatively   A research approach which focuses on meaning that does not use numerical techniques

Quantitatively   A research approach that uses numerical data in observations and measurements

Randomised control trial (RCT)   A research study design that places participants in either a control or an experimental group randomly; a participant has a 50/50 chance of being in either group

Rationalism   All knowledge comes from the mind. René Descartes (1596–1650) stated that mind and matter (body) were separate entities but only humans possessed a mind. This theory was called 'dualism'

Reality   The state of things as they exist

Reasoning   A cognitive process with the aim of understanding or decision-making

Reciprocity   The exchange of things for mutual benefit

Reductionism   Making something as small as can be achieved; separating a person or object into its smallest component parts

Reflection   Involves making a choice to learn from an activity, to learn from our experiences

Reflexive/reflexivity   Capable of 'turning back' on oneself and reconsidering experiences

Reflexive response   Behaviour resulting from rethinking about experiences

Regression   Used in Freud's psychodynamic theory as a mental defence mechanism. It is behaving in a way expected in a previous stage of the lifespan

Reinforcement　A reward or behaviour that supports the re-enactment of a response

Relational ethic　Ethics is making decisions about what is right and wrong; relational ethics is about ethics in relationship with others

Repressing/repression　From psychodynamic theory, a mental defence mechanism that pushes uncomfortable thoughts or feelings into the unconscious mind

Restorative　An approach which facilitates the regaining of equilibrium or sense of well-being

Reticular formation　Nerve pathway in the brainstem influencing the level of consciousness

Reward　A positive reinforcement; a desired thing that is given to a person to recognise achievement and encourage them to do it again

Role model　A person whose behaviour is rewarded and can be imitated

Romantic Naturalists　Philosophers who extol the virtues of nature and biological forces

Satiated　Having a need or desire fulfilled

Schemas　A collection of ideas that together form a conceptual understanding of a thing; a way of managing data or memories

School　A collection of people who think about things in a similar way, or an educational establishment

Self-actualisation　The becoming of oneself, the achievement of one's potential; also called 'peak moments' because it is not a constant state of being

Self-awareness　The extent to which a person knows themself

Self-concept　A collection of thoughts or ideas one has about oneself

Self-disclosure　The sharing of personal information with another person

Self-efficacy　The belief in one's own ability to achieve a goal

Self-evaluate　The judgements one makes about oneself

Self-image　The way one sees oneself; how a person thinks they look

Self-monitors　People who are in a continuous cycle of assessing and managing themselves. As with 'impression management', they use their self-awareness, empathy and social skills to self-regulate by coming alongside others and 'being' what others need and expect of them

Self-perpetuating   Something that continues occurring without an external energy or force

Self-regulate   Where a person monitors and manages their own thoughts, feelings and behaviour

Self-reinforcing or **self-fulfilling prophecy**   Recognising or stating that a thing will happen actually makes it happen

Self-respect   Fostering the practitioner's self-knowledge and care for themself

Self-worth   The value one puts on oneself

Sensitised   As part of behaviourism it is where the organism/person responds to a stimulus more each time it is presented

Serialise   Put items with some similarity into a row, or organise them to occur one after the other

Silo   A way of dividing and separating; to isolate

Similarity   Having things in common

Social learning theory   Learning by observation and imitation; vicarious learning

Social skills   Skills needed to function well in a group

Spirituality   The meaning a person gives to their life

Stable-order principle   Numbers always go in a set order: 1, 2, 3, …

Statistical analysis   A mathematical approach to understanding numerical data

Stigma   The avoidance or mistreatment of a person because they stand out in some way from the major cultural group of the society

Stimulus   Something that provokes a response or action

Stimulus–response theory   A theory that explains behaviour: all behaviour occurs through a trigger or stimulus

Stories   A communicated experience (may be fantasy) with a structure: beginning, middle and end

Storyline   The main theme in a story or the timeline for the story

(The) strange situation   An experiment developed by Mary Ainsworth to assess attachment in infants at about 18 months old

Structuralism/structural theories of personality   A psychological theory that offers an explanation of thoughts and feelings which identified that the structure provides the mechanism for thoughts and is more important than how this is achieved (function)

Subception   From Rogers' theory, this is a term used to identify how people maintain their incongruence. It is where the person deals with an issue without it coming to their direct consciousness; they would then use a mental defence mechanism such as denial to manage the discomfort

Subjective experience   The individual's personal experience

Sublimation   From psychodynamic theory. It is where a thought or feeling that is uncomfortable for the person, usually of a sexual nature, is transformed into a more socially acceptable form such as sport

Substance   Matter, chemical, object

Successive approximation   Through practice, moving behaviour nearer to the desired behaviour – one step building on another

Superego   This is the third part of the personality according to psychodynamic theory. The superego is the part that represents societal rules learned initially through parents

Supervisor   The person who directs or oversees the actions of another

Symbolically   Where something is used to represent something else

Sympathy   To feel for another person

Syntax   The formation of well-constructed sentences

Systematic   A structured process

Systematic desensitisation   'Systematic' refers to a graded introduction to the feared situation, and 'desensitisation' refers to the counter-balancing or reducing of the fear response

Temperament   The natural disposition of the person, which may include their mental, emotional and physical attributes

Temporal   Related to time; present experiences of life in the world

Thanos   Freud's death drive. He suggests that all people are seeking the safety and security of the womb and the only permanent way of achieving this is through death

Therapeutic relationship   With the understanding that 'therapeutic' is to do with offering appropriate treatment, whether this is offering advice or administering medication or activities of daily living. This is a relationship in which therapy can be provided

Timalation   The use of touch to develop well-being

Traits   Stable sources of individual differences that characterise what a person is like

Transactional style   This type of leader performs the role of supervising and organising to gain group performance. Leaders who implement this style focus on specific tasks and use rewards and punishments as motivation

Transductive reasoning   Sees cause where none exists

Transference   From psychodynamic theory; occurs where the client transfers their relational thoughts, feelings and behaviours learned in childhood towards their therapist

Transformational style   These leaders attempt to engage internal motivators, appealing to the person's moral and ethical values; it is more humanistic

Umbrella   A word used to identify a category, a collection of ideas, diagnoses, etc. that have commonalities

Unconditional positive regard   A warm, respectful feeling towards someone without expectation

Unconscious inferences   Ideas that are applied but have not been consciously examined

Unique potential   From humanistic psychology which indicates that each individual is distinct or different: they are unique. Each individual has the ability to achieve certain things: their potential. Hence, 'unique potential' is what an individual is capable of achieving or becoming

Variable   An element that can be manipulated or changed

Vicarious   Learning through observing what happens to another person if they enact a behaviour

Virtue   Used in Erikson's psychosocial developmental theory to mean an ego strength; an achievement of the personality. Also used as an attribute of the personality

Vision   Verb: to sense through sight (eyes); noun: an aim or desire for the future

Index